Dr Sarah Brewer MSc (Nutr Med), MA (Cantab), MB, BChir, RNutr, MBANT, CNHC, qualified from Cambridge University with degrees in natural sciences, medicine and surgery. After working in hospitals and general practice, she realised that many illnesses have a dietary basis, and went on to gain a master's degree in nutritional medicine from the University of Surrey. As well as being a licensed doctor, Sarah is also a registered nutritionist, a registered nutritional therapist and an award-winning health writer. Sarah writes widely on all aspects of health and nutrition, is the author of over sixty popular self-help books and writes regularly for the *Daily Mail*, *Daily Express*, *Daily Telegraph*, and *Prima* magazine. She has found many benefits from using CBD supplements herself.

www.DrSarahBrewer.com
www.twitter.com/DrSarahB

CBD

THE ESSENTIAL GUIDE TO HEALTH AND WELLNESS

DR SARAH BREWER

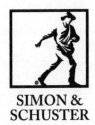

**SIMON &
SCHUSTER**

London · New York · Sydney · Toronto · New Delhi

A CBS COMPANY

First published in Great Britain by Simon & Schuster UK Ltd, 2020

Copyright © Sarah Brewer, 2020

The right of Sarah Brewer to be identified as the author
of this work has been asserted in accordance with
the Copyright, Designs and Patents Act, 1988.

1 3 5 7 9 10 8 6 4 2

Simon & Schuster UK Ltd
1st Floor
222 Gray's Inn Road
London WC1X 8HB

www.simonandschuster.co.uk
www.simonandschuster.com.au
www.simonandschuster.co.in

Simon & Schuster Australia, Sydney
Simon & Schuster India, New Delhi

The author and publishers have made all reasonable efforts
to contact copyright-holders for permission, and apologise
for any omissions or errors in the form of credits given.
Corrections may be made to future printings.

A CIP catalogue record for this book
is available from the British Library

Paperback ISBN: 978-1-4711-9275-3
eBook ISBN: 978-1-4711-9276-0

Typeset in Stone Serif by M Rules
Printed in the UK by CPI Group (UK) Ltd, Croydon, CR0 4YY

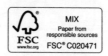

MIX
Paper from
responsible sources
FSC® C020471

Contents

Important Note

This book is for informational purposes only and nothing in it should be construed as medical or legal advice. Information provided is not intended as a substitute for individual medical or legal advice or treatment from your own doctor.

If you are suffering from any health problems, it is important to consult a medical professional before considering medical cannabis or CBD supplements.

While every attempt has been made to verify the information provided, neither the publisher nor the author can accept responsibility for any adverse effects or consequences resulting from the use of any of the preparations or procedures described. Research studies and institutions cited in this book should in no way be construed as endorsing anything in this guide.

1

An Introduction to Cannabidiol

Cannabis is known as the 'plant of a thousand and one molecules' for its treasure trove of biologically active ingredients. The growing recognition of the beneficial effects of these ingredients, alongside changes in legislation, has led to a stampede to cultivate cannabis in what has been dubbed the 'Green Rush' or the 'Big Weed'.

The majority of these newly planted crops are not drug strains of cannabis, however, and have only low levels of THC (tetrahydrocannabinol) – the psychoactive substance that produces the well-known 'high' of marijuana. Instead, large tracts of land are filling with industrial hemp plants that are rich in a wellness molecule known as CBD (cannabidiol).

Word of mouth has quickly spread the powerful message that CBD is a drug-free way to take control of common health problems such as emotional stress, anxiety, sleep difficulties, arthritis and other causes of persistent pain. The new CBD products that have flooded the market are generally viewed as a holistic and effective alternative to marijuana – providing many of the same benefits but without the same altered mental state or 'stoned' effects.

Despite its growing popularity, some people continued to view CBD with suspicion, however, because of its association with cannabis, but this started to change when the World Health Organization (WHO) published a pivotal draft report in 2017. Their Expert Committee on Drug Dependence acknowledged the benefits of cannabidiol for common health issues such as anxiety, chronic pain and insomnia. Importantly, the WHO also confirmed that pure CBD was generally well-tolerated with a good level of safety and no evidence of recreational use or, indeed, any associated public health-related problems.[1] The final WHO Cannabidiol Critical Review Report followed in June 2018, setting the scene for an explosion of interest in CBD and an avalanche of new wellbeing products.[2]

While some people still want the buzz of THC in marijuana, more and more are turning to CBD for its presumed health benefits without the psychoactive 'high'.

Demand for CBD supplements has now grown to overtake sales of vitamin C and the latest estimate is that the global industrial hemp industry will expand from a $4.41 billion market in 2018 to one worth $14.67 billion by 2026.[3] In the UK alone, the CBD market is currently worth £300 million and is predicted to reach almost £1 billion by 2025, according to the Centre for Medicinal Cannabis.[4] All because of a little molecule that was first discovered just eighty years ago.

How CBD was discovered

Cannabis is one of mankind's oldest crops and, during its 6,000 years of use as a source of fibre, food and fuel, our ancestors realised that something present within some cannabis plants could ease pain, aid relaxation and offer benefits for recreational use. When scientists isolated these active components and realised they were unique to cannabis, they became known as cannabinoids to reflect their origin.

The name cannabis comes from the Greek word for hemp, *kannabis*. This in turn is thought to derive from the ancient Sumerian word, *kunibu*, the Assyrian word *qunabu*, or the Scythian word *kanab*. These names may also have given us the Old English word for hemp, *hænep*.

The first known cannabinoid, a mildly psychoactive substance named cannabinol (CNB), was identified over a century ago, in 1896, from a red oil obtained from cannabis resin. Although the resin was known to contain other closely related substances, these were difficult to separate using the methods available at the time. It therefore took another forty years before the next cannabinoid was eventually isolated – this time from hemp plants growing wild in Minnesota, USA.

Researchers led by an American chemist, Roger Adams, harvested the wild hemp after flowering had begun but before the seed had set. Once they obtained their red oil, they treated it to remove the previously identified cannabinol and went on to isolate a new substance which they named cannabidiol or CBD. Announcing their find in the *Journal of the American Chemical Society* on New Year's Day, 1940, they recognised, even at that early stage of research, that CBD was not responsible for the 'high' or 'stoned' effects associated with marijuana.

What gave marijuana its psychoactive effects remained a mystery for another twenty-five years until, in 1964, an Israeli chemist, Raphael Mechoulam, identified tetrahydrocannabinol (THC) as the main mind-bending component of cannabis. The next question was why THC produced these effects, which led to the discovery that we produce our own cannabinoids in our bodies and have our own endocannabinoid system (we will read more about this in chapter three) with which these cannabis extracts interact. To differentiate between these two sources, cannabinoids derived from plants are now referred to as *phytocannabinoids* while those made in the body are termed *endocannabinoids*.

Since then, over a hundred other phytocannabinoids have been identified but the one that is continuing to attract the greatest interest is CBD.

Cannabis research started slowly

Cannabis tinctures and herbal preparations have a long history of use as traditional medicines used to treat a wide range of health problems including pain, infections and convulsions, as well as for general relaxation.

These products fell out of favour when the League of Nations (which existed between the two world wars) was asked to review the negative effects of cannabis resin. Because of its ability to trigger psychotic symptoms in vulnerable individuals, they declared that Indian hemp – an umbrella term for all cannabis plants – should be added to the list of narcotics covered by the International Opium Convention in 1925 and recreational use was banned in participating countries, which included Great Britain. There followed decades of taxation and prohibition designed to restrict cannabis use.

It's now known that different varieties of cannabis plants contain different levels of different phytocannabinoids – no two plants are exactly the same; even those that are cloned and grown under identical conditions will experience slightly different stresses that result in different levels of phytocannabinoids. Cannabis plants with high levels of both THC and CBD are now referred to as drug or marijuana strains, while those with high levels of CBD and only trace levels of THC are known as hemp or, when cultivated to produce fibre and seed oil, as industrial hemp.

During the twentieth century, however, these nuances were poorly understood. The leaves of hemp plants look identical to those of marijuana strains of cannabis. At that time, there was no easy way to distinguish between the two. Both types were known as Indian hemp, although consumers of marijuana products would have noticed that cannabis flowers from some suppliers had significantly different effects to those provided by others.

Things came to a head in 1961 when the United Nations (which evolved from the League of Nations) declared in their Single Convention on Narcotic Drugs that the use of cannabis for anything other than medical and scientific purposes should be discontinued as soon as possible. They further required that, within twenty-five years, all participating countries should adopt measures designed to prevent the misuse of, and illicit traffic in, leaves of the cannabis plant. Not surprisingly, hemp strains of cannabis fell victim to these negative rulings as, even though they contained only traces of THC, this hadn't yet been identified as the psychoactive component of marijuana.

Soon, cannabis was positioned alongside heroin and LSD as a Schedule 1 drug, a classification that is reserved for substances with no accepted medical use and a high potential for abuse. The definition of marijuana in legislation such as the US Controlled Substances Act of 1970 included the resin and all its compounds and derivatives, which automatically encompassed all the cannabinoids, even CBD, regardless of the fact that it is not addictive. Only cannabis stalks, fibre and sterilised seeds were exempted. This made clinical evaluation of the effects of CBD (and THC) in the body of little commercial interest and fraught with legal difficulties.

Research into the beneficial effects of cannabis was reduced to a trickle for many years. Nevertheless, a few inquisitive researchers persevered and, slowly, the therapeutic potential of CBD has emerged from beneath the tarnish of illicit cannabis use.

This early research paved the way for new understandings that differentiated hemp from drug strains of marijuana. It also allowed an evidence-based recognition that CBD has a useful role as a wellbeing supplement that, on its own, is not addictive and has value in treating certain medical conditions.

The number of academic research papers and medical studies involving cannabis has increased year on year from 114 in 1995, to around 2,350 published in 2019 alone.

The health benefits of CBD

I first came across CBD supplements in 2017 when, as a medical writer, I received a press release entitled, 'Britain's Senior Citizens Embrace the Clarifying Benefits of Grannabis'. The term 'grannabis' caught my attention, along with the suggestion that hemp oil extracts were linked with better mental acuity.

The release referred to studies which found that taking cannabidiol extracts reduced the degenerative brain changes associated with Alzheimer's disease, and it quoted a neurology professor who proposed that CBD could potentially slow the progression of dementia for many people.[5]

Strong medical claims such as these have now disappeared as early enthusiasm was quickly stamped on by the Food Standards Agency (FSA), which regulates supplements such as CBD. Classed as a food supplement, CBD can only legally be positioned as having general wellness or nutritional benefits. As soon as CBD manufacturers make a medical claim, they position their product as a medicine and face having it removed from shelves – only products that have gone through extensive (and expensive) clinical trials to prove efficacy and safety are granted licences to claim medical benefits. Even so, most people who use CBD supplements do so not just for wellbeing but to help relieve troublesome physical and emotional symptoms.

Why people use CBD

Unlike THC, CBD has no hallucinogenic or addictive properties but appears to have therapeutic benefits, especially for aiding relaxation, promoting sleep and suppressing the perception of pain.

Between October 2017 and January 2018, an international online survey explored in detail why people choose to use cannabidiol. A total of 2,409 CBD users were recruited (via social media and emails sent to customers by CBD manufacturers) with a fairly equal split between men and women. Most (around 62%) were aged over forty-five years. While nine out of ten respondents lived in the United States, responses were also obtained from people in twenty-three other countries. The survey found that around 38% of respondents used CBD for general health and wellbeing while 62% reported using it to treat a medical condition.[6]

Those taking CBD for medical reasons were, on average, taking it for two or three different conditions, of which the most common were chronic pain, arthritis or joint pain, anxiety, depression, sleep problems and headaches. Half of respondents reported using CBD for less than a year, while one in ten had used it for over five years.

Most people used two different forms of CBD, with sublingual products (sprays, drops or tinctures that go under the tongue) proving the most popular, followed by vaping, capsules and pill forms.

In the United States, a nationally representative survey of 4,355 people in January 2019 estimated that 26% of Americans had tried CBD at least once during the previous twenty-four months – equivalent to 64 million people – while one in seven reported using it every day.[7]

The most common reason for using CBD was to reduce stress or anxiety and aid relaxation. Just under a quarter (24%) reported using it to help with joint pain, 11% for fun or recreation and 10% to promote better sleep.

Overall, one in two people using CBD said it was very or extremely effective. In fact, more than one in five found CBD so effective that they used it to replace their usual medication, including pharmacy painkillers, prescription opioids, anti-anxiety drugs and sleeping pills.

This survey also showed that CBD-infused food or drinks (so-called 'edibles') had overtaken drops, sprays and vaping devices as the most popular way to take it. Following the relatively recent legalisation of medical marijuana by many states in the USA, most people in this survey also said they obtained their CBD from a licensed cannabis dispensary (40%), retail store (34%) or online retailer (27%).

Safety

Perhaps because many people in this survey had obtained their CBD from an official, licensed source, there was a widespread assumption among survey respondents that regulations required CBD to be tested for safety and efficacy by outside labs. Sadly, this is not always the case. While CBD is regarded as safe (as long as you follow the advice in chapter five), some CBD products do not contain the level of CBD stated on the label, some contain more THC than they should and some products have been found to contain contaminants such as pesticides or even synthetic cannabinoids or other drugs – especially those sold online from spurious sources, such as weight-loss aids.

Although the science relating to CBD and other cannabinoids was initially stifled by legislation, so that little research was carried out, this is rapidly changing. Recent research into the health benefits of CBD is starting to support the anecdotal evidence reported in user surveys such as the one above. There is growing evidence that CBD can indeed be effective for a wide variety of conditions, including pain that has not responded well to conventional painkillers. Researchers are also starting to understand that some long-term health conditions may even be caused by faulty functioning of the endocannabinoid system, which may explain why phytocannabinoids (such as those found in CBD products) are helpful for such a diverse range of physical and emotional symptoms.

New research into the benefits of CBD are published almost every day, although many of these studies are carried out on cells grown in a laboratory, or on animals. While this is not ideal, it has provided a firm foundation to support the growing number of clinical studies involving human volunteers. Many of these are small, preliminary studies that aim to confirm that CBD is safe and to better understand what it can and can't do. What is now needed are larger studies to confirm these initial findings.

Never stop taking a prescribed medicine without talking to your doctor first. Always check with a doctor or pharmacist before taking CBD plus a medicine as interactions can occur.

CBD as a food supplement

CBD has only been available in the UK since around 2015. Initially it was bought over the internet and exported from the US, then a few pioneering shops opened that were dedicated to selling hemp-based products. As it slowly became clear that CBD was not just marijuana by another name and that it was legal and here to stay, its use began to grow – mostly through personal recommendation. People who found it helpful as a wellness supplement started sharing their experience with others.

Because CBD is classed as a food supplement, manufacturers are not allowed to make any medical or health claims. That's why labels appear rather stark and do not provide guidance on what conditions CBD can help. User surveys show that most people take it to relieve pain, reduce stress, promote sleep and to generally help them feel more relaxed.

There is still a high degree of official unease relating to CBD because it is derived from cannabis plants – once banned as a source of illegal drugs. This remains the case even when the CBD is derived from hemp and contains only trace levels of the intoxicant THC – nowhere near enough to make you feel 'high'. As a result, the status of cannabidiol (CBD) within different countries is complex and constantly changing.

Up until January 2019, for example, the European Food Safety Authority (EFSA) took the view that only hemp supplements that contained higher levels of cannabinoids than are naturally found in industrial hemp plants were classed as 'novel foods'. This distinction was important because novel foods are defined as those that were not consumed to a significant degree by humans *in the European Union* before 15 May 1997 when the novel foods regulations first came into force. New foods now need to undergo an extensive safety review before they can be sold within the EU – even if they are widely eaten in other parts of the world. Bananas, tomatoes, rice and most spices were once new to our taste buds, for example, and, if introduced now, would be classed as novel foods and first have to pass a full safety evaluation before they could be sold in the EU. Examples of novel foods that have undergone this process and are now on sale in Europe include chia seeds, baobab fruit and krill oil.

As novel foods legislation only mentioned hemp extracts whose cannabinoid concentrations were higher than those naturally found in the plants, manufacturers assumed that supplements whose CBD content reflected the natural concentrations found in hemp were not novel foods. This gave them enough comfort to launch new CBD extracts into the UK market and to invest in promoting their brands as food supplements for general wellbeing.

Then, on 17 January 2019, everything changed. The EFSA quietly amended the entry in the novel foods catalogue to state that all 'Products containing cannabinoids are considered novel foods as a history of consumption has not been demonstrated'. This created panic among CBD sellers as, essentially, the EFSA had concluded that all food supplements containing *any* cannabinoid extracts (including CBD) were novel and, strictly speaking, subject to a full safety evaluation before they could be sold. In effect, all CBD food supplements faced being taken off the shelves until their safety was confirmed – even though the World Health Organization had already stated in their final Cannabidiol Critical Review Report (June 2018) that pure CBD was generally well-tolerated, with no safety concerns or other public health-related problems.

The novel foods regulations are there for good reasons, of course, and are intended to confirm the safety of 'new' foods or new production processes (such as UV-treated mushrooms) before they are sold to the public. It's always possible that a novel food consumed in excess might prove toxic, especially if not prepared properly. One such example was kava kava – a root used in the South Pacific islands to make a tea to soothe anxiety and promote calm. Kava was widely used in Germany for over a century, with shops selling sedative kava tinctures as long ago as the 1890s. These evolved into modern, concentrated tablets and capsules so that higher doses were used than in the traditional infusions used by Pacific Island communities. In 1999, several cases of severe liver damage were associated with kava use in Germany and the US, especially when consumed alongside alcohol and some prescribed drugs. As a result, kava was banned in the UK in 2003.

The novel foods regulations are not legally binding, however, so that individual European Union member states are left to determine the legality of CBD products within their own borders. In practice, most European countries, including the UK, have continued to allow CBD products to be sold in pharmacies, health stores and even supermarkets as long as they do not make medicinal claims and do not contain more than trace levels of THC. However, this may change at any time.

As a full EFSA novel food approval process takes about a year, the UK-based Cannabis Trades Association (CTA) originally decided not to submit a novel foods application for hemp extracts containing CBD to avoid products being withdrawn. Instead, the CTA took the position that cannabis extracts are *not* novel so no approval is needed. The European Industrial Hemp Association (EIHA), for example, has produced evidence that hemp extracts have been used for centuries in the kitchen and as a medicine in both Italy and Germany.

Is Hemp a Novel Food in Europe?
According to the EIHA, the earliest known reference to the medicinal benefits of hemp consumption is inscribed under the Escape Tower on the vault of the Canton de' Fiori in Bologna, dating to around 1220, which reads:

Panis Vita, Canabis Protectio, Vinum Laetitia, which translates as: Bread is Life, Cannabis is Protection, Wine is Joy.

The first cookbook ever printed, *De Honesta Voluptate Et Valetudine* (Rome c.1470), included a recipe for cannabis nectar and mentions using cannabis in wine and cake.

Bruno Laurioux, a chef to Pope Martin V, recommended boiling cannabis flowers and leaves, adding breadcrumbs, onions roasted in olive oil, milk, nuts, raisins, saffron and spices to make a concoction he described as 'good for the infirm'.

Italian medical references mention hemp extracts prepared using fat and honey, distilled water, essential oil, tinctures, alcohol, syrup and liquors.

A cookbook published in 1887 includes a recipe for tortelli pasta, filled with hemp flowers, bacon and cheese.

A less enticing recipe for hemp soup from a German monastery used 6lb of hemp, 3 quarts of wine, white bread, mashed apples, vinegar and spices to produce forty servings.

In February 2020, the FSA announced that all UK CBD manufacturers must apply for a novel foods authorisation for their products by March 2021. While nothing is certain, it is widely believed that CBD will gain EU approval as an authorised novel food, which would allow CBD manufacturers to continue to sell their CBD products, then current uncertainty over whether or not CBD is an authorised food extract will disappear.

IMPORTANT Always check the legality of buying or using any cannabis product (including CBD) in any state or country, and before transporting CBD across any state or national or international borders.

In fact, it's not a good idea to travel with CBD even if you're sure what you are doing is legal, as you can't always expect customs staff at airports to know what it is or know the law, so you may be held up.

While CBD is not a wonder drug, the evidence is building to show that it can help to improve the quality of life for many people who are facing challenges to their physical or emotional health. You can read a summary of this evidence in later chapters.

2

CBD and Medical Marijuana

The versatility of the cannabis plant has given rise to many terms, some of which are used for specific products or in specific ways, and some that are used interchangeably. Not surprisingly, this can cause confusion. Here's a quick explanation of the similarities and differences.

What the terms mean

Cannabis can refer to cannabis plants (whose botanical name is *Cannabis sativa*, see page 74), or to the psychoactive (mind-altering) herbal preparations derived from cannabis plants that are used as recreational or medicinal drugs.

Marijuana, also known as weed, is a popular term for dried parts of the cannabis plant. It is usually made by drying the resinous flowers, buds and leaves of female cannabis plants. The terms *cannabis* and *marijuana* are used more or less interchangeably.

Cannabinoids are a unique group of molecules that were first identified in cannabis plants. These include THC, which causes the 'high' associated with marijuana, and CBD which does not have any intoxicating effects. These plant cannabinoids are also known as *phytocannabinoids* (*phyto* comes from the Greek word *phyton*, meaning 'plant-grown'). It's now known that we also make our own, slightly different cannabinoids in our bodies and these are known as *endocannabinoids* (*endo* comes from the Greek word *endon*, meaning 'internal').

THC (tetrahydrocannabinol) is a phytocannabinoid that causes the 'high' associated with marijuana. High levels of THC are found in marijuana (drug) strains of cannabis plants, while hemp strains have only trace levels of THC.

CBD (cannabidiol) is a plant cannabinoid (phytocannabinoid) that is closely related to THC, but which is non-intoxicating and does not cause a 'high'. CBD is found in good amounts in most types of cannabis plant, whether marijuana strains or hemp strains.

Hemp or **industrial hemp** are strains of cannabis plant that were traditionally used as a source of fibre and oil. They have only low levels of THC but are increasingly grown to obtain the non-intoxicating, wellness molecule, CBD.

Medical cannabis refers to the use of cannabis to help relieve medical conditions such as anxiety or pain. In the UK, doctors who prescribe such products tend to prefer the term *medical cannabis* while people who self-medicate tend to refer to *medical marijuana*.

Medical marijuana is the same as medical cannabis.

Recreational marijuana refers to exactly the same herbal drugs as medical marijuana but when it is used for relaxation or purely to obtain a mind-altering 'high' or 'stoned' effect, rather than to relieve a health condition.

Pharmaceutical cannabinoids are available on prescription in some countries to treat tightly defined medical conditions. These medicinal drugs contain isolated cannabinoid molecules that are either extracted from cannabis plants or synthesised from scratch in a laboratory.

CBD oil is made by combining CBD extract with an oil (such as hemp seed oil, coconut oil or olive oil) to make increasingly popular wellness products.

Hemp oil, hemp extract oil, active hemp oil and similar terms are used to describe CBD oil products in jurisdictions where the legality of CBD is uncertain.

Hemp seed oil is a non-intoxicating and nutritious oil obtained from hemp strains of the cannabis plant (see chapter eight). The pure oil does not contain cannabinoids, but some THC and CBD are often present as a result of contamination from other parts of the plant rubbing up against the seeds.

This book mainly covers the beneficial effects of CBD. While it is increasingly used on its own in a wide range of CBD wellness products, CBD is also an integral part of medical marijuana. In medical marijuana, the ratio of THC to CBD can vary widely.

What is CBD?

CBD is one of at least 113 cannabinoids found in cannabis plants, with some sources claiming that as many as 120 or even 144 exist.[1] In fact, no one knows exactly how many phytocannabinoids there are as some arise only fleetingly as one breaks down into another. New cannabinoids are identified just about every time scientists look, especially when isolated, wild strains of cannabis are discovered in remote parts of the world, or when new advances are made in laboratory techniques.

Cannabinoids present in concentrations greater than 0.5% are relatively easy to find, but those that pass in and out of a brief existence are more elusive. One problem is that fresh cannabis plants contain a different range of cannabinoids during various stages of growth from those present after the plants are harvested, dried and processed.[2]

Within fresh plants, cannabinoids form acidic compounds with tongue-twisting names such as cannabidiolic acid (CBDA) and tetrahydrocannabinolic acid (THCA). CBDA and THCA are closely related to one another as they are both formed from a common precursor called cannabigerolic acid (CBGA). Hemp strains of cannabis plant are genetically programmed to mostly make CBDA, while drug strains of cannabis plant make both CBDA and THCA in varying amounts.

Exposure to air, light or heat triggers these unstable acidic molecules to release carbon dioxide in a reaction known as decarboxylation. This creates more stable, non-acidic molecules: CBDA breaks down into CBD and THCA becomes THC. While the process of decarboxylation mostly occurs during the harvesting and the proper processing of cannabis plants, it also occurs spontaneously within living plants to a certain degree, so that a small amount of CBD is always present during growth and maturation. This is important as when cannabis plants are processed illegally they often contain high levels of CBDA (and THCA) – sometimes referred to as 'raw' CBD (see chapter five on safety). These products will not produce the same beneficial effects as supplements that are processed correctly (at a certain temperature) to convert all CBDA to CBD.

The number and type of cannabinoids present varies between different cannabis strains, different plants within a strain and even within the same plant depending on its age and method of cultivation.

Usually, only three or four cannabinoids are derived from any one plant in significant concentrations, the most common being cannabidiol (CBD) and tetrahydrocannabinol (THC).

THC is a mood-altering, or psychoactive cannabinoid that produces a 'high' – the feelings of euphoria and elation associated with marijuana. THC intensifies and distorts our sensory perceptions, can produce hallucinations and, in some people, can trigger paranoid delusions. THC is also associated with tolerance so that, in the long term, you need to use more and more marijuana to produce the same effects. Using it regularly can also cause withdrawal symptoms. While THC does have medical value as a prescription drug (see chapter six), its recreational use has resulted in the use of marijuana being regulated by law in many countries. Legislation is becoming less prohibitive – even in the UK, which recently authorised certain doctors to prescribe medical cannabis for particular conditions. Medical marijuana is therefore moving more mainstream, as described later in this chapter.

CBD is the most abundant cannabinoid derived from industrial hemp plants and can constitute up to 97% of all the cannabinoids present within the leaves, stems and flowers of cannabis plants. Even in marijuana, CBD is the second most commonly found cannabinoid after THC, accounting for 20 to 40% or more of all the cannabinoids within the plant.

CBD is gaining popularity because, unlike THC, its beneficial effects are not associated with psychoactive or addictive side effects. CBD also blocks some of the unwanted effects of THC within the brain and protects brain cells from damage (in other words, it is neuroprotective). New understandings about the health benefits and safety of CBD mean that its use as a food supplement and as a prescription medicine is increasingly allowed in many countries.

The entourage effect

As well as providing CBD – and THC in marijuana – cannabis plants contain a close family of related cannabinoids, some of which are almost identical to CBD but have slightly different structures that give them slightly different effects. These close relatives include cannabidiol monomethylether (CBDM), cannabidivarin (CBDV), cannabidiorcol (CBD-C1) and cannabidiol-C4 (CBD-C4).

Cannabis plants also contain a rich blend of essential oils. Together, these chemicals naturally protect cannabis plants from ultraviolet light and pests such as bacterial and viral infections. Their odours and bitter flavours also discourage insect attacks and foraging animals.

When used medicinally, these plant cannabinoids and essential oils have a complementary action that is believed to boost the therapeutic benefits of CBD (and THC) in what is known as an entourage effect. This has been likened to the way different musical instruments within an orchestral symphony harmonise the main melody created by the soloists.

CBD in medical marijuana

When drug strains of cannabis plants are used for therapeutic reasons, for example to treat a medical condition such as chronic pain, it is referred to as medical marijuana or medical cannabis (the two terms are interchangeable). Doctors tend to prefer the latter and, in the US, the term 'cannabis' is increasingly preferred. There are concerns that the word 'marijuana' is associated with the idea that cannabis is a harmful intoxicant rather than a herbal medicine. There are also historic racist overtones, which mean some people prefer to avoid it. However, as medical marijuana is the term with which most people are familiar in the UK, I will use it here.

In countries where medical marijuana is legal, prescribed products are usually dispensed as dried, resinous flowers or buds (whole, chopped or powdered) which are eaten or inhaled through a vaporiser that heats the marijuana to a temperature below its combustion point.

Medical marijuana obtained from legal dispensaries or other authorised sources will contain a known quantity of THC and CBD, whose ratio varies. Products with a high THC content have mind-altering (psychoactive) effects such as euphoria, which are commonly described as a 'high' or being 'stoned'. THC also has a downside, however, even when legally authorised, as it can cause side effects such as paranoia, increased anxiety or addiction when used excessively without medical supervision. CBD helps to offset these negative effects of THC in medical marijuana and has beneficial effects of its own in reducing anxiety and promoting relaxation.

It's important to be clear that, even though medical marijuana contains some CBD, it is not the same as CBD supplements that are legally available in health food stores, pharmacies and supermarkets. CBD supplements are derived from industrial hemp – specially bred cannabis plants that are rich in CBD but contain only trace, legal amounts of THC.

The rise and fall of medicinal marijuana

The use of cannabis as a medical therapy dates back at least 5,000 years and probably much longer. The first written reference is credited to the Chinese emperor, Fu Hsi, around 2900 BCE who referred to *ma* (cannabis) as a popular medicine possessing both sacred yin (weak, passive) and yang (strong, active) qualities. In traditional Chinese medicine, these yin-yang qualities are viewed as restoring balance (homeostasis) to an unbalanced body. Around the same time, an ancient text written in Sumerian – one of the earliest languages known – described the use of cannabis to treat seizures.

In 2700 BCE, Emperor Shen Nung, who is revered as the father of Chinese medicine, recognised the psychoactive properties of cannabis in the world's oldest drug encyclo-paedia, the *Shen-nung Pen-ts'ao Ching,* which warned that *ma fen* (cannabis flowers) would produce visions of devils and make you communicate with spirits if taken in excess.

By the turn of the first millennium (1 CE), however, the Chinese pharmacopoeia listed the use of cannabis plants to treat over 100 ailments, including constipation, pain and inflammation. Hua Tuo, the founder of Chinese surgery, even used a compound of cannabis plus wine to anaesthetise patients during surgical operations.

What's in a Name?

- The word marijuana (or marihuana) may derive from the ancient Chinese *ma ren hua*, meaning 'hemp seed flower'. Other theories suggest it is a folk term derived from the Mexican Spanish girl's name, Mari-Juana.
- Marijuana is also known by a long list of slang terms such as weed, pot, grass, herb, bud, budski, ganja, reefer, dope, dak, funk, cheeba, chillum, schwag, wacky baccy, Aunt Mary, Mary Jane, flower tops, gasper, jolly green, joy smoke, yarndi, dutchie, wizard and roach.
- Skunk refers to strong-smelling strains of the cannabis plant that tend to contain high levels of THC.
- *Sinsemilla*, which means 'without seed' in American Spanish, is a potent form of marijuana produced from the flowers of female cannabis plants that are specially tended to ensure they remain unfertilised.

Ancient Egyptians used cannabis to treat inflammation, glaucoma and menstrual cramps, while in India, cannabis was mixed with milk as an anaesthetic and recommended by early Ayurvedic practitioners as a 'cure' for leprosy.

Doctors in ancient Greece and Rome used cannabis to treat earache and other inflammatory conditions, while cannabis roots were boiled in water to ease cramps and joint pain.

In the UK, analysis of fragments of pipe bowls and stems

dating back to Elizabethan times identified cannabis in eight out of twenty-four samples, suggesting that cannabis plants were used alongside the tobacco imported by Sir Francis Drake and Sir Walter Raleigh.

In the seventeenth century, the renowned English herbalist Nicholas Culpeper declared that cannabis extracts could allay inflammations in the head, as well as ease gout, knots in the joints and pain in the sinews and hips. In Victorian times, cannabis tinctures were also used to ease period pains, childbirth, muscle spasms and convulsions caused by tetanus, rabies and epilepsy.

Marijuana was added to the United States Pharmacopeia – a national register of drug information for doctors – in 1854 and tinctures prepared from the flowering tops of 'Indian cannabis' were used to treat muscle spasms, insomnia, neuralgia, vomiting, infections (ranging from tonsillitis to anthrax, cholera, dysentery, typhus and leprosy) as well as seizures, addictions, incontinence, gout, heavy periods and psychoses. So, by the turn of the twentieth century, cannabis was an established, mainstream western medicine. It's thought that the advent of aspirin in 1899 and the invention of the syringe brought an end to its widespread medical use. Injections work faster to relieve pain, but cannabis could not be administered in this way as it is insoluble in water.

The side effects of cannabis, the availability of alternative treatments and the beginning of the US era of prohibition triggered the backlash against this previously popular treatment. In the US, Massachusetts was the first state to declare cannabis illegal, in 1911, and other states quickly followed suit.

Although the dearth of knowledge regarding the medical benefits of marijuana was recognised, only a few scientists were interested in researching its medical benefits. These few were prepared to embrace the legal difficulties to resolve the place of medical cannabis in treating long-term (chronic) conditions. This led to the eventual discovery of THC (tetrahydrocannabinol) as the main psychoactive component of cannabis in 1964 (see page 54).[3] Once the chemical structures of CBD and THC were determined, it became easier to recognise the differences between marijuana, or 'drug strains' of cannabis (with high levels of THC and CBD), and hemp strains (with high levels of CBD but very low levels of psychoactive THC).

Medical marijuana today

Cannabis plants remain the most frequently used, illicit plants in the world, although new legislation is increasingly allowing the use of cannabis for medical purposes. The negative historical connotations of marijuana mean that the cultivation of cannabis plants – even non-drug hemp strains – is still closely regulated. Legal provisions now allow access to medicines containing cannabis via a medical 'recommendation' or prescription in around thirty countries worldwide. According to one estimate, the global market is likely to exceed 55.8 billion US dollars by the year 2025.[4]

Some countries and states have even given the go-ahead for adult *recreational* use of marijuana. This is despite concerns that THC-containing products are potentially harmful for people with existing substance abuse problems, and that regular use may hasten or unmask psychotic illnesses, cause physical dependence and lead to withdrawal symptoms.

This U-turn is partly due to public pressure, partly designed to reduce the drug trafficking that fuels organised crime and partly because of a widespread view that recreational cannabis is less harmful than alcohol when properly regulated.

Medical marijuana in the United Kingdom

Cannabis became illegal to possess, grow, distribute or sell in the UK in 1928, and that continues to be the case for recreational purposes. Until recently, medical marijuana in the form of dried, herbal products were also illegal in the UK. However, high-profile cases and vociferous lobbying have led to medical marijuana becoming legalised in some strictly defined circumstances, although these herbal products are still not easy to access on prescription.

Pharmaceutical Cannabinoids
Pharmaceutical drugs containing cannabinoids have become available in the UK to treat a few specific medical conditions but can only be prescribed by specialists to people who have not responded to other more standard treatments.

The licensed pharmaceutical drugs containing CBD and THC in the form of an oral solution or an oral spray can only be prescribed for a small number of conditions, such as multiple sclerosis and rare forms of epilepsy, as explained more fully later in this chapter. Yet increasing evidence suggests that medical marijuana (in the form of dried herbal preparations) is useful for treating a wide range of other conditions, such as chronic pain.

In October 2018, the chief medical adviser to the UK government wrote to all healthcare professionals confirming that there is conclusive evidence of therapeutic benefit from cannabis-based products for certain medical conditions, and reasonable evidence in several others. As a result, cannabis-derived medicinal products were moved from Schedule 1 of the Misuse of Drugs Regulations (reserved for drugs of no medical use, such as LSD) to Schedule 2 (for drugs with some medical use, such as morphine, but which have the potential for dependence or misuse).

Under this new regime, cannabis-based products (or medical marijuana in the form of dried flowers or resin, for example) are essentially unlicensed medicines, sometimes known as 'specials', and can only be prescribed with rigorous safeguards and auditing, as described below. Interestingly, the new regulations do not restrict how the medicinal cannabis products are taken (whether vaporised, made into a tea, or consumed in food) as long as they aren't smoked (which attracts its own potential health hazards).

When the home secretary announced that doctors in England, Wales and Scotland would be able to prescribe medical marijuana to certain patients from 1 November 2018 campaigners hailed this as a landmark victory. Expectations were high, yet only a handful of patients went on to receive a medical cannabis prescription within the first three months. Of those who did, none were able to fulfil their prescription and actually access their medical cannabis.

Department of Health figures released in September 2019 showed that in the eight months following the introduction of these new regulations, only a very small number of prescriptions for unlicensed 'special' cannabis-based medicines were fulfilled in England.[5]

The difficulty in obtaining unlicensed cannabis-based medicines for legitimate medical reasons is due to several barriers. For example:

- Only doctors who are listed on the Specialist Register of the General Medical Council (which means they are eligible to hold an NHS consultant post) can prescribe unlicensed medical cannabis and only to people with a condition approved for treatment with medical cannabis
- Many specialists are concerned about lack of clinical trials and the lack of evidence on which to balance the risks versus benefits, so are wary of prescribing unlicensed products
- The National Institute for Health and Care Excellence (NICE) has not authorised medical marijuana for use within the NHS because it is not considered a cost-effective use of resources. It may be prescribed by private medical practitioners, however, and private clinics are opening to prescribe medical cannabis where guidelines allow, as described later in this chapter

As a result, many people in England who are unable to obtain medical cannabis on the NHS continue to rely on illegal sources and risk prosecution to obtain their medical marijuana.

In 2005, a nationwide UK survey into the illegal use of cannabis for medical reasons was published in the *International Journal of Clinical Practice*. Out of 2,696 respondents, 25% were using cannabis to alleviate chronic pain, 22% for multiple sclerosis, 22% for depression, 21% for arthritis and 19% for neuropathy. Some were using it for more than one condition.[6]

A more recent national survey of over 10,000 people in England, Wales and Scotland suggests the black market use of medical marijuana is soaring. Commissioned by the Centre for Medicinal Cannabis, the YouGov poll, carried out in October 2019, estimated that 1.4 million people currently use illicit street cannabis for a diagnosed medical problem – equivalent to 2.8% of the adult population. Of these, 56% used it on a daily basis.[7]

This is worrying, because illicit cannabis products contain unknown amounts of THC and CBD – some contain low levels that are ineffective, while others contain high levels that are potentially harmful, especially in products that are concentrated.

Illegal Cannabis Concentrates

Hashish is a cannabis resin traditionally made by collecting the sticky, hair-like glands (trichomes) and 'crystals' found on the outside of cannabis plants. This concentrated source of THC, CBD and other phytocan-nabinoids is consumed by smoking in a pipe, bong or vaporiser. Or it is mixed with herbal cannabis or tobacco and rolled into cigarettes (joints) or cigar wraps (blunts). Other terms for hashish include hash, nup, charas, shish and kif.

Hash oil is a thick, golden brown to black liquid made by grinding cannabis leaves and flowers, adding a solvent, then heating and extracting a sticky gel (oleoresin) under pressure. Hash oil is eaten, smoked, vaped or dabbed (flash-heated and inhaled). The oil is also known as honey oil, cannabis oil, wax, shatter, budder and butane hash.

Rosin is made in a similar way to hash oil, but without the solvent – a combination of heat and pressure is used to squeeze the resinous sap from the plant.

While dried cannabis flowers typically provide between 10 and 25% THC, hashish can contain as much as 65% THC and hash oil up to 90% THC by weight.

Private clinics in the UK

While the NHS does not currently consider medical mar-ijuana to be a cost-effective treatment, obtaining it is becoming easier for those who are able to pay.

A national medical cannabis registry was launched in November 2019 to build the body of evidence needed to support NHS prescribing and convince policymakers that medical cannabis should become as widely available as other treatments for those who would benefit from it.[8] The registry aims to recruit 20,000 patients to gather real-world evidence on the effectiveness, safety, quality-of-life and medical outcomes of prescribed medical cannabis. Initially, it will focus on seven conditions that are believed to respond to treatment with cannabinoids and will enrol patients for whom other treatments have failed. The seven conditions selected for initial study include three physical conditions (chronic pain, epilepsy and multiple sclerosis) as well as four mental health conditions (post-traumatic stress disorder, Tourette's syndrome, anxiety disorder and substance use disorder). Treatment will be provided at a network of clinics across the UK which will prescribe medical cannabis at an 'affordable', subsidised cost. To find out how to enrol, visit drugscience.org.uk/project-twenty21.

These legal, private clinics are staffed by consultants who specialise in prescribing medical cannabis and have been set up to help overcome the barriers that, until now, have limited patient access to this newly authorised medical treatment. They work within tightly controlled limits approved by all relevant regulatory authorities so every prescription is agreed by a multidisciplinary team and signed off by their medical director as appropriate. The medical cannabis products prescribed all have known levels of THC and CBD.

Cannabis law is in a state of flux and likely to change in the UK and the rest of the world. The information provided here and below is only correct at the time of writing – do check the current status in your country before using medical marijuana or taking CBD supplements.

Medical marijuana elsewhere in the world

Within **Europe**, the availability of medical marijuana varies according to country. While smoking marijuana is the traditional mode of recreational use, no EU country currently authorises the smoking of cannabis for medical purposes as inhaling smoke from burning plants exposes users to harmful tars and other particles. Where medical marijuana is available on prescription, it is obtained from authorised dispensaries that provide dried cannabis flowers (called buds, which are dispensed whole, chopped or powdered) for vaping or making tea.

The Netherlands (which is famous for its laxity towards recreational cannabis), Germany, Italy, Norway, Denmark and Finland, for example, have all now given the green light to medical marijuana on prescription.

Uruguay merits a mention as it became the first country in the world to legalise recreational marijuana (alongside medical marijuana) in 2013. No products were available for sale in authorised pharmacies until 2017, however, as it took this long to put robust regulatory systems in place. The marijuana sachets provided in pharmacies in Uruguay are restricted to a relatively low potency of 2% THC balanced by 5% or 7% CBD. Customers have to register with the regulator and purchases are limited to 10 grams a week (using fingerprints to prove identity) to encourage moderate use.

In the **United States**, medical marijuana was illegal throughout the country until 1995. In 1996, California became the first state to allow the medical use of marijuana with a doctor's recommendation. Fast forward to December 2019, and medical marijuana is legal in thirty-three out of fifty states and the District of Columbia, with legalisation pending in a further fifteen states.

In addition, some states have passed laws that only allow the use of high CBD/low THC products for medical reasons in limited situations. Recreational marijuana is also legal in eleven states and DC (for adults over the age of twenty-one) although it continues to be fully illegal in others.

Confusingly, however, marijuana remains illegal at the federal level for any purpose as it is still classified as a Schedule 1 substance under the Controlled Substances Act (1970), which makes the distribution of marijuana a federal offence. Federal law also prohibits doctors from prescribing marijuana, so doctors can only write a *recommendation* for medical marijuana, rather than a prescription. Furthermore, federal law bans the interstate transport of marijuana so it is illegal to carry it across state lines – even between states in which marijuana is legal and when it has been legally obtained. In any case, most states have only legalised locally grown marijuana produced to specific state standards and sold by licensed local suppliers.

In states that have chosen to legalise cannabis (for recreational or medical use) the maximum level of THC allowed is typically below 0.3%, but individual regulations vary between states from zero to 0.8%, 3% and even 5% THC (with at least an equal amount of CBD).[10] There are also limits on the amount you can possess and you may need to join a patient registry or carry a medical marijuana card or personal licence.

In May 2018, over 2.1 million people were registered for a medical cannabis identification card across the thirty-three states with legalised medical cannabis.[11] Chronic pain accounts for around 65% of qualifying conditions for medical cannabis use in the US; other conditions include multiple sclerosis, cancer and irritable bowel syndrome.

Canada has allowed the use of marijuana for medical purposes since 2001. The recreational use of marijuana was also legalised in October 2018 – only the second country to do so after Uruguay. Strict laws are in place, however, that aim to allow adults access to cannabis while, at the same time, keeping it out of the hands of youths and stopping criminals from profiting.

For medical use, those authorised by their doctor can buy cannabis directly from a federally licensed seller by registering with Health Canada – the government department responsible for overseeing public health and medical drugs. Individuals can also grow a limited amount of cannabis for their own medical use or designate someone to produce it for them, although the amount you are allowed to possess is restricted unless you are authorised to obtain cannabis for medical purposes when higher amounts may be prescribed.

In October 2019, the cannabis regulations also allowed the legal production and sale of three new classes of cannabis product that can be used for recreational or medical use in Canada: edibles (e.g. gummies, chocolate, non-alcoholic drinks, baked goods), extracts (e.g. oil for vaping) and topicals (e.g. ointments, oils and makeup).

Australia continues to ban the recreational use of marijuana. Federal law has permitted medical marijuana since 2016, although its legality varies according to state. In Victoria, for example, medical cannabis is only permitted for children with severe forms of epilepsy; New South Wales will consider medical marijuana for adults with a terminal illness, while Queensland suggests that medicinal cannabis may be suitable for treating a wider range of serious health issues (e.g. severe muscular spasms and other symptoms of multiple sclerosis, chemotherapy-induced nausea and vomiting, some types of severe epilepsy, palliative care and some forms of chronic non-cancer pain). In these cases, authorised doctors can apply to prescribe cannabis in a variety of forms, including seeds, extracts, resins, tinctures, vapes, capsules, oils or sprays.

New Zealand made cannabis illegal in 1927, but an amendment to this legislation in 2016 allowed doctors to prescribe approved pharmaceutical cannabinoid drugs. Further legislation, introduced in December 2017, has paved the way for the introduction of a Medical Cannabis Scheme that will establish a medicinal cannabis agency and a licensing regime to widen access. A yes/no referendum is also planned for 2020 so that New Zealanders can vote on whether or not cannabis should be legalised for sale in licensed premises or for limited home cultivation.

Cannabis and CBD regulations are in a state of flux world-wide. It is important to check the legal status of CBD in your country/region/state before buying and before taking it with you when travelling abroad.

Information on the legality of medical marijuana in different countries and US states is available from marijuanadoctors.com/international-patients

---

Potential side effects of medical marijuana

Like all drugs, medical marijuana can have side effects. Those most commonly reported include fatigue, sleepiness, dizziness, nausea, changes in appetite, dry mouth, feelings of euphoria (intense happiness) or depression, confusion and, occasionally, hallucinations or paranoid delusions, psychosis or cognitive distortion (untrue thoughts).

The extent of side effects varies with the concentration of THC and whether or not a significant amount of CBD is present to help balance these unwanted effects.

The main concerns with using *recreational* marijuana is that it appears to increase the risk of developing a psychotic disorder in some people – especially if THC levels are high and CBD levels are low. This is especially likely in illicit street forms of the drug whose high strength is intended to create a 'stoned' effect. Prescribed forms of medical marijuana reduce these risks by providing a known amount of THC that is balanced by a known amount of CBD.

A study published in the *Lancet Psychiatry* in 2019, for example, found that daily marijuana use was associated with a 3.2-fold increased risk of a psychotic disorder compared with those who had never used marijuana. This rose to nearly a five times increased risk in people using highly potent forms of marijuana.[12]

Preliminary studies presented at an American Heart Association scientific meeting in November 2019 also found that young people who frequently use marijuana (more than ten days a month) were nearly 2.5 times more likely to have a stroke compared to those not using it. And people who are addicted to marijuana are also 50% more likely to be hospitalised for a serious heart rhythm abnormality than those who don't use marijuana.[13] These risks may remain the same whether you use marijuana for recreational or medical purposes, although prescribed products provided by licensed dispensaries are likely to be safer as they provide a known (and usually relatively low) level of THC, which is balanced by a known level of CBD.

If using medicinal or recreational cannabis, it is important not to drive or operate machinery due to the risk of experiencing drowsiness. Always check for interactions with any prescribed or over-the-counter drugs you are taking. There is a good interactions checker at Drugs.com.

CBD in the UK

To ensure the required low levels of THC, manufacturers within Europe are only allowed to produce CBD from the stems and leaves of industrial hemp plants (not the flowers) and these plants must be tested before harvest to prove they contain no more than 0.2% THC (although this level may increase in future). In addition, CBD products may only be sold as a nutritional supplement if they contain less than 1mg THC in total *per pack*, whatever its size (not per dose). Any CBD product that contains *more than* 1mg THC in total is therefore illegal.

The maximum permitted level of CBD in industrial hemp plants grown in the European Union is under review. The 0.2% cut-off currently allowed may be increased to match the level allowed in the US and Canada (0.3%), or even to 1% to match that allowed in neighbouring Switzerland.

CBD in the rest of the world

Regulations relating to CBD vary widely from country to country. In some, its sale is freely allowed with no restrictions, while in others it remains illegal.

The **United States** has seen an upsurge in popularity of CBD. In 2018, the so-called Farm Bill made cultivation of industrial hemp federally legal as long as plants are grown by a licensed producer and contain no more than 0.3% THC (by dry weight). As a result, the US hemp industry grew from virtual non-existence into a $1 billion market by 2018 and, according to the *Hemp Business Journal*, sales will likely reach $1.9 billion by 2022.[14] Of this, hemp-based CBD products are expected to account for $646 million.[15]

However, the US Food and Drug Administration (FDA), which oversees food supplements, initially took the view that, even though hemp cultivation was now legal, CBD products were not, based on their interpretation of existing laws. This didn't stop hundreds of CBD products coming to market as the FDA appeared to favour a flexible approach with 'a light touch' and 'enforcement discretion' to recognise the change in federal law on hemp. In practice, they

The Cannabis family includes many closely related plants including hemp and marijuana strains

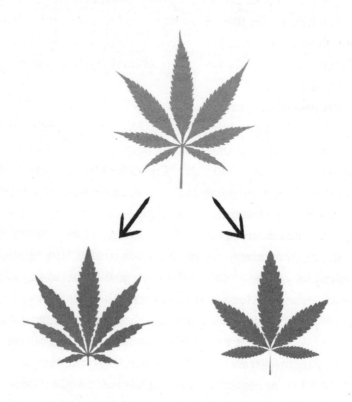

Hemp strains of Cannabis are used as a source of fibre and CBD

Marijuana strains of Cannabis are grown for their high levels of THC

Even though hemp contains low levels of THC, it also contains higher levels of other beneficial cannabinoids (such as CBD) which may promote relaxation and calming effects in the body.

decided not to challenge manufacturers except when flagrant medical claims were made.

Even so, in June 2019, the state of Massachusetts decided to crack down on the sale of CBD products and prohibited any food containing hemp-derived CBD, including hemp dietary supplements and even animal feeds containing hemp products.

Because of the confusion over the legal status of CBD in the United States and the vast array of products flooding the market, four trade groups sent an open letter to all senators urging Congress to pass timely legislation clarifying that hemp-derived CBD products (i.e., not obtained from marijuana strains of cannabis) are lawful as long as they meet appropriate quality and safety standards.

In the meantime, many manufacturers in the United States are playing it safe and choose not to mention CBD on labels at all. Instead, they describe their CBD products using terms such as 'full strength hemp oil', 'therapeutic hemp oil', '20% hemp oil', 'active hemp', '2,000mg hemp', 'strong hemp extract', 'hemp oil extract' or 'premium hemp drops'. This makes it difficult to know exactly what you are buying – a hemp seed oil extracted from hemp seeds (which, while nutritious, contains very little CBD) or a CBD-rich extract from resinous hemp flowers that is then mixed with a carrier such as hemp seed oil to make a true CBD oil.

By the time you read this book, the status of CBD supplements in the US should be more transparent, if not crystal clear.

In **Canada**, the Canadian Cannabis Act that legalised cannabis in 2018 also regulates other plant cannabinoids, including CBD. Products containing CBD must be derived from hemp plants that contain no more than 0.3% THC and can only be legally bought with a prescription from an authorised cannabis retailer for medicinal use or from a legal recreational outlet.

Australia does not allow the recreational use of CBD and it is not available as a food supplement. CBD is only available legally in Australia from an authorised prescriber to treat a small number of specific medical conditions, such as rare forms of severe epilepsy. In July 2018, the Australian government increased access to CBD through the Special Access Scheme. This allows doctors in certain states and territories to register to prescribe medical CBD products to certain patients.

New Zealand no longer classes CBD as a controlled drug but as a prescription medicine as long as the amount of THC present does not exceed 2% of the total CBD content. As with all medicines, it can only be obtained on prescription from a doctor.

Out of the 195 recognised sovereign countries in the world, at the time of writing, around fifty now allow the sale of hemp-derived CBD supplements, including Bulgaria, the UK, the Netherlands, Germany, Cyprus, Czech Republic, Greece and South Africa. It still remains either strictly illegal or only available on prescription in the other countries, however, so always check before taking CBD with you when travelling.

Pharmaceutical cannabinoid drugs

Some licensed pharmaceutical drugs contain cannabinoids. These are not the same as medical marijuana (made from dried cannabis flowers) or CBD supplements (made from hemp). Instead, these pharmaceutical drugs contain concentrated amounts of cannabinoids that are either extracted and purified from cannabis plants or made artificially in a laboratory. If synthetic, the cannabinoids may be chemically identical to the CBD or THC found in cannabis plants or may be entirely new molecules not found in nature, but they have effects in the body that are similar (and often more powerful).

They are manufactured to pharmaceutical standards to provide a known amount of cannabinoids in every dose. In order to have gained their pharmaceutical licence, they need to have undertaken supporting, good quality, clinical trials that show evidence of effectiveness in treating particular health conditions and acceptable safety when balancing their benefits against their potential risks.

Licensed cannabinoid drugs are only authorised for use by prescribing doctors to treat specific medical conditions and only in certain situations. Typically, they can only be prescribed by specialist doctors when treating a patient in whom other, first-line medical treatments have failed.

A number of cannabinoid drugs have been developed, but what is available on prescription differs from country to country.

Illegal Synthetic Cannabinoid Drugs

Beware: some forms of cannabis, often with exotic-sounding names, contain herbs (not necessarily marijuana) sprayed or mixed with synthetic cannabinoid drugs (aminoalkylindoles).

While these narcotics mimic the effects of cannabis, some are fifty to 100 times more potent. They can cause toxic side effects including abnormal heart rhythms, seizures, kidney failure, liver damage, severe bleeding (when laced with warfarin rat poison), psychosis and even respiratory failure. They have been linked with several deaths, especially when mixed with other recreational drugs or alcohol.

New synthetic psychoactive substances may be sold online legally until authorities catch up, identify them and specifically classify that particular chemical as illegal.

Hundreds of synthetic cannabinoids have been identified and buying 'spice' products on the internet has been likened to playing chemical Russian roulette – sooner or later you are likely to encounter a lethal combination.

CBD as a pharmaceutical drug

While cannabis plants contain a blend of over one hundred different cannabinoids, including THC and CBD, a prescription-only drug is now available that contains virtually pure CBD extracted from cannabis plants.

This pharmaceutical CBD drug is currently licensed to treat seizures associated with two rare and severe forms of epilepsy: Lennox-Gastaut syndrome and Dravet syndrome, both of which start in childhood and are associated with frequent, daily seizures that are difficult to control with standard anti-epilepsy drugs.

The exact way in which the pharmaceutical doses of CBD reduce seizures is unknown, but is believed to result from an ability to damp down overexcited neurons.

Clinical trials involving around 1,500 patients show that these pharmaceutical CBD drugs help around one in three people with Dravet syndrome to become seizure free, while in others the number of seizures is reduced by treatment.[16]

The use of these pharmaceutical CBD medicines is strictly regulated. In the UK, for example, specialist doctors can only prescribe them to patients aged two years or over, must check the frequency of convulsions every six months, and stop treatment if the frequency of seizures has not fallen by at least 30% compared with the six months before starting treatment.

Important: someone with epilepsy should only take a CBD supplement or any form of medical marijuana if their doctor agrees, and close supervision is vital. Interactions can occur with other anti-epilepsy medications which may reduce their effectiveness or increase the risk of unwanted side effects. It's also important to know that medicines bought online can be illegal versions that contain counterfeit and potentially unsafe drugs. If you decide to purchase medications online (which I don't recommend but do consult your own doctor), be sure you are buying from a reputable, properly accredited online pharmacy.

The dose of prescribed CBD drugs is much higher than when taken as a food supplement. Even so, most people taking them do not experience the potential side effects. Those listed in the patient leaflet provided with the medication as most common include drowsiness, decreased appetite, diarrhoea, fever, feeling tired and vomiting. Potentially serious side effects that doctors monitor their patients for include changes in liver enzyme levels and, less commonly, suicidal thoughts – if you experience any of these tell your doctor immediately.

Suicidal Thoughts

Contact your doctor immediately if you have thoughts about suicide or dying. You can also find help via:

UK: Samaritans, samaritans.org. Tel: 116 123 around the clock, twenty-four hours a day, 365 days a year.

Befrienders Worldwide: find your country's helpline at www.befrienders.org.

Interactions

CBD has the potential to interact with many prescribed and herbal medicines. Always check for interactions via your doctor or pharmacist. If they are unable to help, there is a useful interactions checker at Drugs.com.

CBD plus THC in pharmaceutical drugs

A prescription-only oral spray that contains THC and CBD extracted from cannabis plants is available with the generic name of nabiximols. Nabiximols is mainly prescribed to treat multiple sclerosis (MS) although the licence varies slightly by country.

Each depression of the spray delivers almost equal parts THC to CBD – the CBD is added to help reduce the psycho-active effects of THC and to improve its tolerability.

The exact way in which nabiximols reduces spasticity and pain is not fully understood. It is believed to interact with the human endocannabinoid system (see page 52) to improve limb mobility and to reduce the perception of pain. It is also undergoing clinical trials for potential use in severe neuropathic cancer pain.

Synthetic pharmaceutical cannabinoid drugs

A few pharmaceutical drugs that contain synthetic cannab-inoids are available for prescription in limited situations. These synthetic drugs tend to mimic the effects of THC and are therefore very different to CBD. Because they can cause addiction and withdrawal symptoms with long-term use, they are only prescribed for short periods of time to treat serious health conditions such as nausea and vomiting during cancer chemotherapy.

Where cannabinoid research is going

Cannabinoids – whether natural or synthetic – are an exciting area of research, especially as it's now thought that some long-term health problems are associated with changes in the levels of endocannabinoids that we make ourselves. This is explained more fully in the next chapter, but drugs that can mimic or block our own endocannabinoids are now seen as a potential answer to many conditions that are currently difficult to treat, such as pain due to nerve damage, fibromyalgia, migraine and irritable bowel syndrome.

Synthetic cannabinoids that mimic the effects of CBD on the immune system are already in development to reduce inflammation. These drugs are currently being investigated for potential use in autoimmune and inflammatory diseases such as systemic sclerosis (scleroderma), dermatomyositis and cystic fibrosis.

Caution is needed, however, based on the experience with rimonabant, the generic name for a synthetic cannabinoid drug that was launched in Europe in 2006 to suppress appetite and promote weight reduction in obesity. While it worked well in helping people lose weight, it was withdrawn in January 2009 due to adverse psychiatric effects such as increased anxiety, depression, and suicidal thoughts.[17]

Unsurprisingly, researchers and doctors alike want to ensure that new cannabinoid drugs are not launched until their potential for serious side effects is fully assessed.

In summary, the medicinal use of cannabis plant

extracts has now come full circle, from its traditional use as a healing therapy, through a period of prohibition and back to increasing acceptance as an effective medical treatment.

3

CBD and the Endocannabinoid System

The reason why CBD, THC and pharmaceutical cannabinoid drugs have an effect in the body is because we make at least five closely related, but different, cannabinoids ourselves. Known as endocannabinoids, they interact with special proteins found on and inside our cells that are known as cannabinoid receptors. These receptors act rather like the whiskers on a cat to detect signals – in this case the presence of a cannabinoid molecule (whether one we've made ourselves, or one obtained from cannabis plants). Activation of these cannabinoid receptors acts as a trigger that produces a change in that cell. For example, making the cell less active, so fewer pain messages are passed on. Other cells may respond by becoming more active and increasing their output of hormones. In other cases, receptor activation may lead to the production of protective substances that make the cell less susceptible to damage when oxygen levels are low.

Together, our endocannabinoids, their receptors and the enzymes needed to make and recycle them form our endocannabinoid system (ECS).

The endocannabinoid system is an ancient communication network that first appeared within the animal kingdom millions of years ago to control feeding responses. In hydra, for example, the tiny, freshwater creatures with many tentacles, endocannabinoids regulate the opening and closing of the mouth when food is detected. Something similar still controls suckling in human babies and the way we respond to the sight and smell of food.

Researchers now recognise the ECS as one of our most important regulatory networks, helping to maintain a balanced state (known medically as homeostasis), including the harmonious interactions that occur between our central nervous system (brain and spinal cord) and our peripheral nerves, internal organs, hormone-secreting endocrine glands and immune cells.

The ECS therefore helps to regulate almost every important human emotional and physical function including our appetite, mood, sleep, memory, immunity and our responses to stress and pain. It is involved in controlling fat and energy metabolism as well as reproduction and even the life cycle of our cells. Endocannabinoids also allow our brain cells to communicate in ways that aid our learning, memory and our ability to think straight (cognition).

In 1998, researchers reviewing the endocannabinoid system summed up the messages it produces as 'relax, eat, sleep, forget and protect'.[1]

Most of the beneficial effects of CBD are due to its ability to mimic or support the effects of our own endocannabinoids, acting as a messenger to help maintain all these delicate body balances controlled by the endocannabinoid system.

How the endocannabinoid system was discovered

Despite its antiquity, the ECS was only discovered relatively recently. In the 1960s, Israeli chemist Raphael Mechoulam wondered why marijuana was able to trigger a high. It was already known how other recreational drugs, such as opium and cocaine, produced psychoactive 'stoned' effects, but exactly how marijuana worked remained a mystery.

While the existence of CBD had been known since 1940, Mechoulam was the first to isolate THC and recognise its psychoactive potential in 1964. Mechoulam was also the first person to start using the term 'cannabinoids'.

THC and CBD are produced within cannabis plants from a common parent molecule, cannabigerolic acid (CBGA), so it's not surprising that their molecular structures are very similar. It is the seemingly small differences between the two, however, that result in CBD having such different effects to THC in the body.

Both CBD and THC are fat soluble and easily cross the blood–brain barrier to reach the central nervous system. Initially, it was assumed that they exerted their effects by 'numbing' brain cell membranes in a similar way to general anaesthetics. It was only when synthetic cannabinoids were labelled with a radioactive form of hydrogen that researchers were able to trace exactly how these molecules interacted with brain cells. This led to the discovery of our specific cannabinoid receptors to which CBD and THC were 'sticking'. The first cannabinoid receptor was identified in 1988 and the second in 1993. These receptors were dubbed CB1 and CB2.

The fact that we have these cannabinoid receptors caused researchers to scratch their heads – they obviously weren't there on the off chance that our ancestors happened to consume cannabis. Logically, they must have specific functions in the body and we must have internal chemicals with which they naturally interact. This led to the discovery of our own endocannabinoids which, although different to those found in cannabis plants, share close structural similarities. The first endocannabinoid, with the clumsy chemical name of N-arachidonoylethanolamide, was isolated in 1992 and became known as anandamide after the Sanskrit word *ananda*, meaning 'bliss' or 'supreme joy', due to its uplifting effects on mood.

Bliss describes the happiness that creates body and mind harmony. Ananda was a principal disciple of the Buddha and, in Buddhism, the name also indicates an elevated consciousness.

A second endocannabinoid, 2-arachidonoylglycerol (2-AG), was reported in 1995,[2] followed by three other endocannabinoids (named noladin ether, virodhamine and N-arachidonoyl-dopamine or NADA), though we don't yet fully understand what they do.

Cannabinoid receptors

Although we only have two main types of cannabinoid receptor, we each own billions, if not trillions of them. Some are embedded within the outer membranes of our cells, while some are found inside cell compartments and anchored to the cell nucleus.

CB1 receptors are mainly located within the central nervous system (brain and spinal cord) and are involved in regulating brain cell activity. They are especially concentrated in the areas of the brain responsible for memory, cognition (ability to think straight), emotion and co-ordination. Outside of the brain, CB1 receptors have been found within nerve endings, immune cells, the gut, heart, lungs, liver, kidneys, bladder, bones, reproductive organs, eggs, sperm and embryos, eyes, adrenal glands, thyroid gland, pituitary gland, skin and several types of cancer cells. The fact that CB1 receptors are present in so many different locations led researchers to suspect that our endocannabinoid system is more important for general health than was previously realised.

Activation of CB1 receptors causes the 'high' associated with marijuana.

The type of CB1 receptor you inherit may determine your susceptibility to the negative effects of THC, and your risk of becoming dependent on marijuana.

CB2 receptors are mainly concentrated within the immune system, where they regulate our immune responses and inflammatory reactions. Some CB2 receptors are also found in the brain, especially in scavenger cells called microglia, which act like cleaners – clearing up cell debris and pruning away unwanted neural connections. The number of CB2 receptors in the brain increases when we experience long-term pain or suffer from neurodegenerative diseases such as Alzheimer's and multiple sclerosis. CB2 receptors appear to regulate how nerve cells grow, divide and survive. Outside of the brain, they are concentrated in immune tissues such as the lining of our intestine, the spleen, tonsils and thymus gland (which is found behind the sternum and programmes a type of immune cell known as T-cells). CB2 receptors are also found in the heart and bloodstream, liver, fat cells, bone and the reproductive system, including eggs, sperm and embryos.

In fact, it's now believed that cannabinoid receptors are present in virtually every cell type and play a critical role in maintaining balance throughout the body. This balance helps to bring cell activity and the level of important chemicals (such as salts and hormones) back towards the normal range if they start to become too high or too low.

CB1, CB2 – and CB3?

A receptor called GPR55 is another candidate for membership of the endocannabinoid system and appears to be involved in regulating inflammation and pain. There are calls for GPR55 to be relabelled as the CB3 receptor.

Two other cannabinoid receptors, known as the WIN receptor and the abnormal-cannabidiol (abn-CBD), have also been identified but their function remains uncertain.

Each cannabinoid receptor consists of a protein – a long chain of amino acids – that is folded into a complex, three-dimensional shape and winds in and out of cell membranes seven times.

The 3D structure of CB1 receptors was first published in 2016 and that of the CB2 receptor only recently, in 2019. Their structures are very similar, but it's the differences that allow them to interact with different cannabinoids in different ways to produce potentially opposite effects in what has been described as a yin-yang relationship.

When a cannabinoid receptor detects an endocannabinoid (or a plant cannabinoid if you are taking CBD or medical marijuana) it changes shape. This acts as a switch that triggers a response within the cell, either increasing or suppressing certain activities such as immune reactions, to help bring the body back into balance and restore wellness. It is thought that cannabinoid receptors located on nuclear membranes may even be involved in switching certain genes on or off as needed to help cells adapt to changing situations.

The way a cannabinoid receptor responds to an endocannabinoid can be different to the way it responds to a phytocannabinoid or to a synthetic, pharmaceutical cannabinoid drug. This is because the slight chemical and structural differences between the human, plant and man-made molecules affect how they lock onto the receptors. Some lock on to trigger a big change in the receptor shape, some create a partial response, while others may block the receptor altogether so it can no longer work. CBD only weakly activates CB2 receptors, for example, and is thought to produce many of its beneficial effects via other types of receptor and by reducing the breakdown of our own endocannabinoids (so they can act for longer). In contrast, THC locks onto CB1 receptors to create stronger feelings of euphoria (the marijuana 'high') than are achieved by our own endocannabinoids.

Backward signalling

Within the brain, nerve cells (neurons) are separated by a narrow communication gap called a synapse. Information is mostly transmitted across these gaps by communication chemicals called neurotransmitters, which usually only travel in one direction across the gaps. This ensures that messages only pass along set pathways linking one brain cell to the next to prevent information chaos. However, it was long suspected that some form of reverse chemical transmission was possible – even essential – to help damp down overactive states.

In an exciting advance in 2001, our two main endo-cannabinoids were identified as the elusive molecules that are able to travel backwards across some types of brain cell synapses. The direction in which they travel in any particular synapse depends on which side of the gap the endocannabinoid is made and released. In other words, the endocannabinoid system is able to pass messages against the normal flow of information within the brain (a process known as retrograde synaptic signalling). This allows the endocannabinoid system to pass messages back down the line to suppress overexcitable brain cells and stop them from releasing new neurotransmitters into the synapse. Researchers have found that this suppression can last for as long as 'tens of seconds'[3] – an astonishing length of time given that a nerve can send up to 1,000 impulses per second, which means that it is likely to have profound importance in regulating brain activity.

These new understandings have led to the theory that faulty functioning of the endocannabinoid system and endocannabinoid deficiencies may be implicated in some long-term health problems such as depression, chronic pain syndromes and neurological diseases, as we will read later.

Importantly, it may also explain some of the benefits of CBD in helping to suppress a wide range of conditions associated with brain overactivity such as anxiety, pain, sleep difficulties and some forms of epileptic seizures.

How CBD interacts with the endocannabinoid system

In biochemistry, a molecule that blocks a receptor so that it cannot function properly is known as an antagonist (or blocker), while a molecule that activates a receptor to produce a biological response is known as an agonist.

To make things more complicated, different agonists have different levels of activity. Some fully activate a particular receptor to produce the maximum response and are known as full agonists. Some only partially increase the activity of a receptor and, unsurprisingly, are known as partial agonists.

There are also substances that can bind to a receptor but produce the opposite effect to a full agonist. These are known as inverse agonists. For example, a pharmaceutical cannabinoid may act as a full agonist on cannabinoid CB1

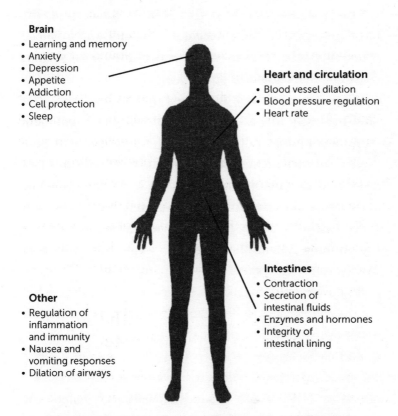

Brain
- Learning and memory
- Anxiety
- Depression
- Appetite
- Addiction
- Cell protection
- Sleep

Heart and circulation
- Blood vessel dilation
- Blood pressure regulation
- Heart rate

Intestines
- Contraction
- Secretion of intestinal fluids
- Enzymes and hormones
- Integrity of intestinal lining

Other
- Regulation of inflammation and immunity
- Nausea and vomiting responses
- Dilation of airways

Widespread Effects of Cannabinoids in the Body

receptors to cause major agitation, another cannabinoid (such as THC) may act as a partial agonist on the same receptors to cause less severe anxiety, while a third plant cannabinoid (such as CBD) may act as an inverse agonist on that receptor to have the opposite effect and cause relaxation. These different effects help to explain the differing actions of the plant cannabinoids, CBD and THC, although their effects are not yet fully understood despite several decades of research.

THC partially activates both CB1 and CB2 receptors but has a greater effect on CB1 receptors. This accounts for most, if not all, of the psychoactive effects of marijuana such as euphoria, hallucinations and anxiety.

When it was initially discovered that, unlike THC, CBD only modestly interacts with either type of cannabinoid receptor and does not activate CB1 receptors to create a 'high', early researchers rather ignored CBD because of its lack of exciting marijuana-like effects. It was only when its anti-seizure and anti-anxiety effects were recognised, followed by the discovery that CBD had beneficial effects on the immune system, that researchers started to look more closely at how it worked.

It's now known that, with CB1 receptors, CBD creates the opposite effect to THC by generating calm and damping down overstimulation and anxiety – in other words, it acts as an inverse agonist. The fact that CBD does not directly stimulate CB1 means it does not produce the same 'stoned' effects as THC. It also means that CBD can reduce the unwanted side effects of THC (such as anxiety, sedation, psychosis, hunger and rapid heartbeat) to improve its safety. Recently, scientists discovered that CBD does this by altering the shape of the CB1 receptor so that THC cannot gain access to stimulate the receptor as well as it usually does.

With CB2 receptors, CBD also acts as an inverse agonist, which may partly explain how it helps to reverse the effects of inflammation.

The way cannabinoids interact with CB1 and CB2 receptors is complex, however, and, besides their independent functions, CB1 and CB2 receptors also appear to work together in some cases, causing each other to respond in unexpected ways.

These complicated interactions may help to explain the so-called entourage effect (see page 23) in which the other plant cannabinoids present within hemp plants help to boost the beneficial effects of CBD. These additional cannabinoids are believed to provide a more 'rounded' CBD supplement that works better for reducing anxiety and pain than a more pure CBD supplement (often described as a narrow-spectrum or CBD isolate supplement, as described in chapter five).

Cannabidiol works in many different ways

It was soon realised that CBD has more widespread effects than can be explained by its weak interactions with CB1 and CB2 receptors alone, however. Scientists therefore started to look at other ways in which it might work, and were surprised to find so many.

CBD is now known to interact with at least sixty-five different types of cell receptor, which helps to explain why it has such a wide range of beneficial effects.

Most of the evidence suggests that, within the nervous system, CBD enhances the action of our own main endocannabinoid, anandamide, slowing its reabsorption and breakdown after it is released. In this way, CBD prolongs the natural, uplifting 'blissful' effects of anandamide which, as described earlier, can act as a reverse signal to damp down overactive brain pathways. This interaction may partly explain how CBD produces such a rapid calming and relaxing effect.

Other effects of CBD that are believed to result from its ability to prolong the effects of anandamide range from dilating blood vessels (to lower body temperature and blood pressure), to suppressing pain and regulating the way our immune system naturally prunes away abnormal and worn-out cells.

CBD can also act on non-cannabinoid receptors to cause levels of calcium to increase within certain cells. This may add to the pain-relieving and anti-inflammatory effects of CBD, as well as helping healthy cells to survive when oxygen levels are low. For example, studies suggest that CBD may restore normal calcium levels in brain cells that are not functioning properly, which may help to protect against some neurological diseases. As calcium acts as a signal for the release of neurotransmitters and the contraction of muscles, this may also explain how CBD helps to suppress some forms of epileptic seizure.

One of the most exciting effects of CBD is its ability to block an important immune substance known as TNF-alpha (tumour necrosis factor-alpha), which has been shown in laboratory studies involving human white blood cells.[4] TNF-alpha acts as a powerful trigger for inflammation and its overactivity is implicated in many serious inflammatory diseases such as rheumatoid arthritis, plaque psoriasis and Crohn's bowel disease. While still under investigation, these new understandings are helping to focus the direction of future cannabinoid research in the hope of developing CBD-based treatments.

Turmeric spice also blocks the production of TNF-alpha, giving the combination of CBD plus turmeric great potential for treating pain associated with inflammation.

Other receptors with which CBD can interact include serotonin receptors (to lift mood and produce 'feel-good' effects), inhibitory receptors which have a calming effect on our central nervous system, as well as other receptors that are involved in pain, stress responses and cell communication. Through all these interactions, CBD helps to support and maintain normal conditions within the body, including the brain.

CBD may also work to reduce pain in a similar way to aspirin by suppressing enzymes that produce prostaglandins – hormone-like chemicals that are involved in triggering inflammation, pain and fever.

CBD also appears to have strong antimicrobial activity against fungi, viruses and bacteria, including against so-called superbugs such as MRSA.[5]

CBD is an antioxidant

On top of all the above, CBD is a powerful antioxidant and mops up harmful free radicals, suppressing inflammation and pain. A free radical is a molecular fragment that carries a spare electrical charge which makes it highly unstable. Free radicals damage cells in a process known as oxidation, which is similar to the chemical reaction that turns iron into rust. Cells are constantly under attack from free radicals and this oxidative stress contributes to premature cell ageing and, when genetic material is damaged, can cause mutations that result in cancer.

We can't escape free radicals altogether, as they are generated by normal cell metabolism (such as the production of energy), but their number greatly increases in people who smoke, are exposed to pollutants or who have raised blood glucose levels (diabetes).

As an antioxidant, CBD neutralises free radicals and helps to protect cells – especially brain neurons – from degeneration caused, for example, by low oxygen levels, nutrient deficiencies, inflammation and abnormal build-ups of protein.[6]

Comparing the effects of CBD and THC

The many different interactions between CBD and different classes of receptor in the body mean that it produces a different range of actions to THC, and has different effects on our emotions (see chapter seven) and physical health (see chapter six). The fact that CBD is not psychoactive (does not cause a 'high'), is not addictive and does not cause withdrawal symptoms makes CBD a more useful phytocannabinoid than THC as its benefits are not marred by these unwanted side effects.

The following table shows some of the important ways in which the actions of CBD and THC differ and ways in which they are similar.

Action	CBD	THC
Psychoactive (produces a 'high')	✗	✓
Addictive potential	✗	✓
Withdrawal symptoms	✗	✓
Prolongs the effects of anandamide	✓	✗
Reduces anxiety	✓	✓/✗*
Antipsychotic	✓	✗
Anticonvulsant	✓	✗
Sedative	✓	✓
Reduces pain	✓	✓
Protects brain cells from damage	✓	✓
Lowers blood pressure	✓	✓

* THC reduces anxiety at low doses but can cause anxiety in higher doses and in those who have not taken it before.

Conditions linked with low endocannabinoid levels

When there is a proven endocannabinoid deficiency, taking a supplement that contains CBD is believed to help restore equilibrium within the endocannabinoid system and to have beneficial effects in a wide range of conditions. It's likely that, in the near future, more prescription-only forms of CBD and other cannabinoids will become available to treat an even greater range of conditions. There is growing evidence that deficiencies within the endocannabinoid system could be involved in many common health problems, including anxiety, stress, pain and inflammation.

The world's first cannabidiol tablet containing pure CBD in fixed doses is already in development in the Netherlands for use as a pharmaceutical drug to treat neurological diseases.[7]

No other internal regulating system discovered during recent years has raised as many expectations for the development of new life-enhancing and life-extending treatments. Drugs that activate cannabinoid receptors (agonists) or which block their effects (antagonists) are currently being sought as future pharmaceutical drugs.

Drugs that target CB1 receptors (which are concentrated within the central nervous system) are likely to help manage pain, reduce inflammation, treat obesity and substance addictions, as long as they do not have unwanted psychological effects like those associated with marijuana.

Drugs that target CB2 receptors (which are concentrated within immune cells) have the potential to treat autoimmune conditions (in which the immune system wrongly attacks parts of the body, such as rheumatoid arthritis); conditions in which excess scar tissue is formed (fibrotic conditions such as scleroderma); pain due to nerve damage (neuropathic pain) and diseases associated with the destruction of nerve cells (neurodegenerative diseases such as Alzheimer's and Parkinson's disease). Some evidence even suggests that blocking CB2 receptors may suppress tumour growth as future cancer treatments, although these suggestions are far from proven.

New studies to explore the full potential of CBD are underway globally with one in ten of them taking place in the UK.[8]

CBD products sold as food supplements are not allowed to make medical or therapeutic claims, so they are styled as a wellbeing supplement to support general relaxation.

Based on the World Health Organization's review of cannabidiol, published in June 2018, and other reviews highlighting conditions that may involve deficiencies within the endocannabinoid system, pharmaceutical CBD drugs may have therapeutic benefits in a surprisingly wide range of conditions which are summarised in the table below.

Medical conditions that may benefit from new CBD-based therapies

Addictions

Alzheimer's disease

Anxiety

Arthritis (all forms, including osteoarthritis, rheumatoid arthritis, psoriatic arthritis and gout)

Attention deficit hyperactivity disorder (ADHD)

Cancers (including bladder, leukaemia, prostate,
   lung, thyroid, breast, glioblastoma (a type of
   brain cancer)
Cardiovascular diseases
Chronic constipation
Chronic obstructive pulmonary disease (COPD,
   including chronic bronchitis and emphysema)
Chronic pain
Depression
Diabetes and diabetes complications
Diverticular disease
Eczema
Epilepsy
Huntington's disease
Hypoxia-ischemia injury (cell damage due to low
   oxygen levels)
Infection
Inflammatory diseases (e.g. Crohn's disease)
Insomnia
Irritable bowel syndrome
Liver failure
Malaria
Multiple sclerosis
Nausea
Obesity
Obsessive compulsive disorder (OCD)
Pain
Parkinson's disease

Post-traumatic stress disorder (PTSD)

Psoriasis

Psychosis (e.g. schizophrenia)

Rheumatoid arthritis

Stroke

Tinnitus

As yet, there is not enough evidence from human clinical trials to confirm all these uses. However, the research findings relating to CBD and medical marijuana in some of these conditions are explored later in this book.

What about other phytocannabinoids?

While most clinical studies have concentrated on the effects of CBD and THC and their interactions with the endocannabinoid system, the other phytocannabinoids and essential oils found in CBD extracts and in medical marijuana are widely believed to have synergistic actions that enhance one another as part of the entourage effect. Some examples of the additional cannabinoids found in cannabis plants include:

Cannabichromene (CBC), which has anti-inflammatory, sedative, analgesic, antibacterial and antifungal properties and helps to block pain and inflammation.

Cannabidivarin (CBDV), which helps to prevent epileptic seizures.

Cannabigerol (CBG), which has some anti-cancer properties and is also antibiotic.

Cannabinol (CBN), which is formed from the breakdown of THC and is also a legally controlled drug. It is half as active on CB1 (psychoactive) receptors but three times more active on CB2 receptors than THC. Like CBD, it therefore affects the immune system more than the central nervous system.

Tetrahydrocannabivarin (THCV) which has been identified as a potential appetite suppressant that may be useful for treating obesity and diabetes.

How to support your own endocannabinoid system

If you are feeling stressed and in need of relaxation, or if you are anxious or in pain, your endocannabinoid system is likely to be working harder than normal and may become less effective. Taking a CBD supplement may help to boost the effects of your own endocannabinoids so they are better able to bring your body back into balance.

User surveys show that many people find CBD helps to relieve a wide range of physical and emotional conditions. Everyone is different, however, and the genes we inherit (which provide the blueprint for making our own endo-cannabinoids and their receptors) mean we may respond to supplements in different ways. Because CBD has such a wide range of actions, however, it is likely to provide some benefit for most people as it interacts with the body in at least sixty-five different ways. In comparison, conventional painkillers such as aspirin or paracetamol have more limited ways of working and, as a result, around one in three people do not respond to their analgesic effects (see page 127).

Some people may respond best to a CBD supplement that is labelled as 'full-spectrum' as this contains the full range of phytocannabinoids found in hemp plants, including trace levels of THC. Others may respond better to a CBD supplement labelled as 'broad-spectrum' as this has had all the trace amounts of THC removed. Yet others may do best with a relatively pure CBD supplement that has had all the other cannabinoids removed – these are labelled as 'narrow-spectrum'.

The majority of people will not notice a difference between the different types, but if you do not achieve the result you were looking for by taking one type of CBD supplement, it is worth trying another blend.

Before taking CBD supplements, however, read chapter five on how to use them safely.

4

How Hemp Is Grown for CBD

Classification of the cannabis plant family is controversial but three main species are broadly identified.

Cannabis sativa, the form now largely cultivated in the West, can grow tall – up to 4.5 metres – and has distinctive leaves with long, thin blades. Sativa plants have high levels of CBD and varying levels of THC, ranging from low to high depending on the strain.

Cannabis indica is a 'wild' species from India that naturally forms short, bushy plants with broad-bladed leaves. Indica plants tend to have more equal amounts of THC and CBD and are said to have more relaxing and sedating properties than sativa plants. Indica strains are often favoured for indoor growing as they are smaller and bloom earlier than sativa plants.

Cannabis ruderalis, first identified in Russia, forms short, weedy plants with thin stems and leaves that have fewer blades. These generally contain high levels of CBD and low levels of THC.

This botanical classification remains uncertain, however, as these species readily cross-pollinate to produce fertile hybrids, such as the so-called *Cannabis afghanica*, which is believed to have originated from a cross between sativa and indica strains.

Because of the ability of all cannabis plants to interbreed, some botanists argue there is really only one species, with many subspecies, referred to as *Cannabis sativa* L. (the 'L.' stands for Linnaeus, the Swedish botanist who first named the species).

To make things more complicated, cultivation and selective breeding over hundreds of years have also led to the development of many different strains (or cultivars) of cannabis plants that contain different blends of cannabinoids and aromatic essential oils. This selective breeding has resulted in hemp strains – with high levels of CBD and very low levels of THC – being cultivated primarily for fibre, seeds and recently CBD supplements and marijuana strains – with generally high levels of both CBD and THC – as a source of medicines.

The Legal Definition

Since 1961, international law has defined the cannabis plant as 'any plant of the genus *Cannabis*' in order to cover *Cannabis sativa*, *Cannabis indica* and *Cannabis ruderalis* plus any new varieties discovered in the future.[1]

'Strains', 'varieties' and 'cultivars'

The terms 'variety', 'cultivar' and 'strain' tend to be used synonymously to describe a group of plants that have descended from a common ancestor and share characteristics.

'Cultivar' is a contraction of 'cultivated variety' and refers to a group of cultivated plants that have been bred to share the same uniform characteristics (such as high CBD, low THC). The seed-grown offspring of these plants usually have the same characteristics as the parent plants (although random mutations can occur).

'Variety' is a less specific term for plants that are not necessarily cultivated, and can refer to both naturally occurring wild types as well as cultivated plants.

'Strain' is the term used most widely by cannabis breeders. It refers to plants that have descended from one particular parent with a particular characteristic (e.g. colour, scent, relaxing effects). The seed-grown offspring of these plants may not necessarily have the same characteristics as the parent plants and the desired characteristic may only be replicated by cloning. Breeders name their cannabis strains to emphasise the distinctive qualities of their products, such as smell or taste, to differentiate them from others on the market.

There are over 600 named, modern varieties or strains of cannabis plant. Some contain more CBD than THC and some the reverse, while others contain a more balanced blend.

In most countries where hemp farming is legal, only seed from certified varieties of cannabis plants can be marketed or grown. In the EU, for example, around seventy types are included in the catalogue of plant species that are permitted to be grown. In the US, each state has its own list of permitted and prohibited varieties of hemp plant.

What's in a Name?
Cannabis plants are commonly called industrial hemp when used as a source of fibre, hemp seed when used as a source of seed oil, phytocannabinoid-rich (PCR) or CBD-rich hemp when used to produce CBD, and marijuana when used as a source of therapeutic or recreational psychoactive drugs.

The scent of cannabis

In addition to the 120 or so cannabinoids present in cannabis plants, there are also around 140 different types of essential oils which readily evaporate to release a detectable smell. These all contribute to the odour, taste, colour and medicinal properties of different marijuana strains.

Some of these aromatic substances, such as pinene, camphene, myrcene and limonene, are also found in other resinous plants such as pine trees, mint and citrus peel, and give different cannabis products a strikingly distinctive scent. These aromas and flavours are judged in marijuana competitions in a similar way to those that assess wine, coffee and beer.

Can You Smell Cannabis?
Some people are unable to smell cannabis. The reason why is not fully understood but is most likely a genetic quirk, like how some people can't smell asparagus while others can't

smell musk. This may be a specific form of 'smell blindness' in the olfactory system similar to colour blindness in vision.

Connoisseurs claim they can tell just from the smell of a cannabis product whether or not it has medicinal effects and the strength of the associated 'high'. In an interesting study published in 2018,[2] sixty-one volunteers were asked to sniff dried cannabis flowers obtained for recreational use from licensed dispensaries – no touching, smoking or eating was allowed. Eleven cannabis strains were assessed blindly, with two included twice to check for sniff consistency, making thirteen samples in all.

Each volunteer was placed in a well-ventilated room. They were presented with a wide-mouthed, amber glass bottle that contained 1g of dried cannabis flowers from one of the samples, in random order. After sniffing the sample, they were asked to place a tick against all the scents they detected from an alphabetical list of forty-eight different smells associated with marijuana.

The top ten most frequently identified scents were earthy, herbal, woody, flowery, sweet, citrus, pungent, pine, tea and sage.

When volunteers were asked which samples they thought were most potent, those in the citrus group won out. These were also thought to be of higher quality and to have a higher perceived price. However, while the researchers found a 3.5-fold difference in concentration between the sample with the most THC and that with the least, the level of THC did not correspond to any particular scent profile or to volunteers' estimate of potency based on smell alone. This just goes to demonstrate that you can't tell the strength of a CBD extract or medical marijuana based on just their scent, which is not surprising given that pure THC and CBD are odourless. Filtered CBD oils that are clear and smell less pungent can be just as effective at alleviating your symptoms as those that make you screw up your nose.

Plant selection is reducing levels of CBD in marijuana

Because users of marijuana are usually looking for a 'high', some growers have cross-bred different varieties of cannabis plant to produce new strains with increased levels of THC to produce the strongest 'stoned' effects.

THC is concentrated within the female flowers and resin-producing hair-like glands (trichomes) that grow among the flowers. As well as selective breeding, growers also discovered that, if they ensured female flowers remained unfertilised, their cannabis plants would put all their energy into producing large, cannabinoid-rich flowers instead of seeds. As a result, over the last thirty years, marijuana products have increasingly contained more and more THC and less and less CBD to balance out its effects.

Sinsemilla, which means 'without seed', is a potent form of marijuana produced from the flowers of female cannabis plants that are specially tended to ensure they remain unfertilised.

Levels of THC in *sinsemilla* are at least twice that of normal cannabis and up to ten times higher as a result of the carefully controlled environmental conditions provided for hydroponically grown plants, depending on the strain.

In the 1980s, marijuana plants typically provided a final THC content of 3% (dried weight). When scientists analysed 38,681 illicit cannabis products (mostly dried flowers) seized by US drug enforcement agents over a period of twenty years, the results were surprising. The average THC content rose from 4% in 1995 to at least 12% in 2014 in the United States. At the same time, levels of CBD in marijuana dramatically reduced, changing the ratio of THC to CBD from around 14:1 in 1995 to over 80:1 in 2014. As a result, illegally obtained marijuana is now more potent than ever before and there is too little CBD to help balance its effects. When high levels of THC are not balanced by CBD the risk of side effects, such as aggression, paranoia, memory loss, poor co-ordination, difficulty thinking straight and addiction, greatly increases. As a result, visits to hospital emergency departments for health problems and accidents involving marijuana have increased over time alongside its potency.

The same thing has happened in Europe. The average potency of marijuana samples analysed in 2015 had THC levels that were 80% higher than those sampled in 2006, and 90% higher for cannabis resin (which is made by collecting the sticky secretions found on the outside of cannabis plants). The range was still wide, however, with concentrations of

THC in marijuana in the EU varying from 3 to 22%, while in the resin samples THC levels went from 4 to 28%.[3]

A THC level greater than 1% in a cannabis extract can have enough of a psychoactive effect to produce a 'high'.

Growing hemp

Hemp is the umbrella term for non-drug strains of the cannabis plant. These fast-growing, flowering annuals have been cultivated for thousands of years for a variety of uses. Their long, leggy stems provide woody and absorbent fibres that were traditionally used to make rope, paper, textiles and clothing, as well as pet bedding. Our ancestors also valued hemp seeds as a nutritional food and used their oil as lamp fuel.

The earliest archaeological finding of hemp fibre used to make cord dates back 12,000 years to a Neolithic site in China. Within the British Isles, the first mention of hemp was around 373 BCE, when a Celtic princess with the memorable name of Cambri Formosa championed the use of hemp for weaving and sewing among her clanswomen.

By the sixteenth century, hemp plants were so essential for making naval ships' sails, rigging, ropes, haulage sacks and sailors' uniforms that King Henry VIII passed a law in 1533 forcing farmers to grow a certain amount of hemp or flax. For every 60 acres farmed, they were required to set aside 1 rood (about a quarter of an acre) for hemp or flax or face a hefty fine of three shillings and four pence – the equivalent of half a year's wages for a typical servant. Hemp became so valuable that farmers even used it to pay their taxes in place of coin.

The wide cultivation of hemp throughout Europe and Scandinavia is revealed in the number of place names containing the word 'hemp', 'hamp' or 'henef', such as Hampshire, Hempstead and Hempnall Green in England, Hempriggs in Scotland and Hennef in Germany.

Once metal replaced the wood in ships, however, and cheaper fibres such as abacá (sometimes known as Manila hemp, derived from a species of banana plant), jute and cotton became more widely available, the hemp industry started to wane.

Slave labour in America reduced the price of cotton and its softer feel made it preferable to hemp for producing textiles in the UK.

Following a sixty-five-year hiatus between 1928 and 1993 when hemp growing was illegal in the UK, it is now enjoying a revival. In fact, industrial hemp is the ultimate, multi-purpose crop. It supplies fibre and hemp seed oil (which can be added to skincare products or consumed as a nutritious food) and is used to make concrete-like building materials, paint and even biodegradable plastics which are stronger yet lighter than polypropylene.

It is increasingly viewed as a sustainable resource that is helping to reduce our dependence on petrochemicals such as petroleum oil and natural gas. For example, the hemp biomass (plant material left behind after the fibre is stripped out) can be decomposed in a reactor to produce an oil that can be used for fuel – every dry ton of biomass produces as much as 80 gallons of renewable gasoline – or a charcoal-like product that can be used as an organic fertiliser.

Increasingly, however, hemp plants are being specifically selected, bred and cultivated as a rich source of CBD.

Growing hemp for CBD

Even though it's now legal to grow hemp in the UK, it's still mandatory to apply for a Home Office licence and follow strict regulations. Only approved strains of hemp plants can be grown commercially (not for personal use) to produce CBD. These are *Cannabis sativa* strains that have a high cannabidiol content but low THC levels (less than 0.2% total cannabinoids). The exact strains and the parts of the plant that may be processed are strictly regulated.

Currently, within the UK, CBD destined for food supplements may only be derived from the mature stalks of certified strains of industrial hemp. Some other countries allow CBD for supplements to be obtained from the leaves and even the flowers, which have a significantly higher cannabinoid content.

Male and female plants

Cannabis plants are dioecious, which means they mostly exist as separate males, which produce pollen, and females, which produce seed. In some cases, however, female plants can be forced to produce pollen sacs as well.

Farmers growing hemp for fibre may select male plants for their height, harvesting them before they are fully mature for maximum strength. But if growing hemp to produce hemp seed, you need female plants and a few males to produce the pollen to fertilise them.

Cannabis pollen is wind-borne and just one or two pollen-producing plants can fertilise a whole field of female cannabis plants. As soon as a female plant receives pollen it ceases to flower and puts all its energy into producing seed rather than cannabinoids. So if the hemp is being grown for CBD, pollination would make plants less commercially attractive. In regions where it is legal to extract CBD from hemp flowers (rather than just from the stems, as in the UK), farmers want cannabis plants that produce lots of flowers and cannabinoid-rich, resinous glands (trichomes). However, they don't want any seeds at all, and must ensure pollination does not occur by shunning male cannabis plants and only growing cloned female plants or sowing *feminised* seed.

Feminised Seed

A mature female plant near the end of its life cycle can be stressed (e.g. by changing the temperature, light conditions, soil acidity or spraying plants with a silver solution). This triggers the production of female pollen sacs as a survival mechanism to allow self-fertilisation.

Female pollen lacks male chromosomes and, when used to pollinate other female plants, results in feminised seeds which only produce female offspring.

How hemp is cultivated

It is illegal to grow hemp plants in the UK without a licence, so don't be tempted to do this at home! Other countries and states have different legislation, as mentioned in chapter two.

Hemp Is a Self-offsetting Crop

Industrial hemp absorbs more carbon dioxide per hectare than any forest or other commercial crop. It's estimated that 1 ton of harvested hemp fibre absorbs around 1.6 tons of carbon dioxide.[4] What's more, this CO_2 is permanently bonded within the fibre meaning it cannot escape back into the environment.

Hemp plants are considered a very easy crop to grow. Not only does hemp grow extraordinarily rapidly, with some strains reaching 4 metres in as little as 100 days, their fast growth and leafy canopy suppress weeds, meaning herbicides aren't needed, while their natural protection against fungi, bacteria, viruses and insects makes pesticides often unnecessary. As a result, many crops are certified as organic and this makes them an attractive crop for organic farmers and environmentalists. Hemp fibres also have a natural antimicrobial resistance which makes them long-lasting.

Hemp can thrive in most environments except extreme deserts and high mountains. It grows best at temperatures of between 15°C and 27°C, in a moderately humid atmosphere and with 50–80 centimetres (20–30 inches) of rain during the growth cycle. Strains bred in Europe tend to flower prematurely when planted in hotter climes such as Australia, so each country has its own preferred varieties.

Hemp puts out a well-developed root system that prevents soil erosion and needs less water than other fibre crops, such as cotton, which makes it suitable to grow in dry regions with irrigation.

Decontamination

Hemp soaks up contaminants and is used to cleanse soils in a process known as phytoremediation. Hemp was planted in Chernobyl following the nuclear disaster, for example, to remove radioactive waste and heavy metals such as caesium, strontium, cadmium, chromium and lead. The hemp plants can then be used to produce clean fibre while the contaminated parts are incinerated to catch the radioactive ash.

When grown to produce fibre, hemp is planted close together to promote long, thin, leggy stems and to discourage branching and flowering. When grown for CBD extraction, however, plants are allowed more space to promote leafy growth. In regions where it is legal to process the flowers for CBD, hemp is planted further apart to encourage bushy growth and abundant flowers.

Great care is needed when cultivating hemp for CBD as anything that stresses the plants – such as drought, flooding, heat, cold or even nutrient excesses or deficiencies – will cause THC levels to spike to protect the plant. This is known colloquially as 'going hot' and, if THC levels exceed permitted cut-offs, it means the plants are no longer legally classified as hemp but as marijuana and may have to be destroyed.

Similarly, if it is the hemp flowers that are to be used (rather than just the stems and/or leaves), close vigilance is required to weed out any rogue plants bearing pollen sacs (male or female). Just one plant could wind-pollinate the whole crop, triggering seed production and reducing the CBD concentration.

Hemp-free CBD?

Scientists writing in the journal *Nature* have found a way to produce cannabinoids from the simple sugar galactose using yeast cultures that are genetically engineered to produce CBD or THC by inserting cannabis genes.[5]

Harvesting hemp

Industrial hemp that is grown for fibre or CBD production from the stalks is harvested as soon as the last pollen is shed but before the seeds have set; this is usually between ten and fourteen weeks after planting. If the crop is destined to be made into CBD products, the exact date is determined by testing to ensure levels of THC are below the cut-off required to classify the crop as hemp and to maximise CBD levels as much as possible. Hemp plants grown for fibre are typically 10–15 feet tall when harvested.

Hemp grown for seed is harvested later, around sixteen to eighteen weeks after planting, when around three quarters of the seed has ripened and birds are starting to strip them from the plants. Seeds at the top of the head are less mature than those at the bottom, so if farmers wait too long, the bottom seeds will start to shed (known as shattering). Hemp strains grown for seed are typically 6–9 feet tall when harvested.

Once harvested – sometimes by hand using machetes rather than machines – the hemp plants are hauled indoors for drying in well-ventilated conditions.

In all cases, local laws will determine what happens to the parts of the hemp plants not used to produce fibre, seed or CBD. In the UK, for example, a Home Office licence is needed to grow low-THC cannabis plants to produce hemp fibre for industrial use, or to extract hemp seed oil. The green parts of the plants – the resinous flowers, buds and leaves, which are the parts of the plant that are controlled – must be destroyed after harvesting, with only the fibre, mature stalks or seeds allowed to leave the premises. Additional licences are needed to use other parts of the plant to produce CBD as a food supplement or for research or medical use.

Current Legislation Is Wasteful

The fact that the green parts of the plant must be destroyed rather than used for other manufacturing purposes is a shame. According to the British Hemp Association, hemp plants have over 10,000 potential industrial applications, ranging from plant protein and food supplements through to bioplastics, biofuels, construction materials and textiles.

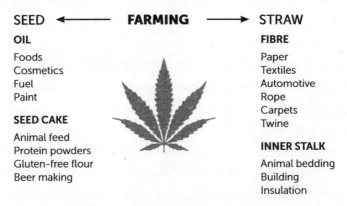

SEED ◄——— **FARMING** ———► STRAW

OIL

Foods
Cosmetics
Fuel
Paint

SEED CAKE

Animal feed
Protein powders
Gluten-free flour
Beer making

FIBRE

Paper
Textiles
Automotive
Rope
Carpets
Twine

INNER STALK

Animal bedding
Building
Insulation

Potential Industrial Uses of Hemp

There is much disquiet over the legal restrictions that limit the potential uses of hemp and prevent growers from processing the whole plant. With the global movement towards creating sustainable, environmentally responsible products, these restrictions are in need of a sensible review.

Growing hemp in the rest of the world

Laws relating to the cultivation of cannabis plants are under scrutiny and likely to change in the future. The information provided here is only correct at the time of writing – do check the current status in your country as they are subject to change.

In the **United States** hemp was set to become a billion-dollar crop until the Marijuana Tax Act of 1937. This failed to differentiate hemp from drug strains of cannabis plants and effectively made the cultivation of industrial hemp illegal. This was repealed during the Hemp for Victory campaign in the Second World War, when fibre was needed to make rope for the US Navy, but was then re-enacted once hostilities ended.

In 1970, Schedule 1 of the Controlled Substances Act banned the growing of cannabis plants of any kind, including hemp. Schedule 1 is the highest level of control reserved for substances that are deemed to have no safe medical use and which carry a high risk of being abused or misused. Pilot programmes to study hemp were only allowed under strict licence for limited purposes such as medical research.

Colorado became the first US state to legalise industrial hemp in 2012 for producing fibre and oil. In 2018, the Agriculture Improvement Act (commonly known as the Farm Bill) allowed hemp cultivation by licensed producers, according to federal regulations, as long as plants contained no more than 0.3% THC (dry weight). The Farm Bill removed low-THC CBD products from the definition of marijuana but did not make them legal at a federal level (see chapter two). Additional licences are needed to extract CBD and, even then, if a bumper crop bursts through the 0.3% THC limit when harvested, it legally becomes marijuana and must be destroyed.

Within the **European Union** (and currently reflected in the UK), only approved seed varieties can be planted and, at the time of writing, industrial hemp must contain no more than 0.2% THC when harvested.

When THC limits were first set in 1984, the permitted level was 0.5%. This was reduced to 0.3% three years later and, in 1999, further reduced to 0.2% because of concerns about the harmful effects of THC. An amendment to increase permitted

THC concentrations back up to 0.3% has now been approved by the European Parliament Committee on Agriculture and Rural Development. If this receives authorisation and is passed into law, the higher level may come into effect in 2021.

In **Australia**, the 1937 ban on growing hemp was overturned in April 2017 so that industrial hemp can be grown under a licence issued by a state government. According to the National Farmers' Federation, hemp is now grown in every Australian state to produce seeds, oil, fibre or woody inner stalk (hurd/shiv).

Hemp plants must contain low levels of THC, which varies by state.

Farmers in **New Zealand** require a licence to grow hemp as an agricultural crop. The varieties of *Cannabis sativa* grown must have a THC content below 0.35%. However, industrial hemp products cannot be used for creating therapeutic products such as CBD, which requires separate licensing. CBD is currently classified as a prescription-only medicine in New Zealand.

Canada legalised the growing of industrial hemp in 1998. Farmers must obtain a licence and may only plant certified seeds from authorised cultivars approved as having less than 0.3% THC levels.

Extracting CBD from hemp

CBD is present in most above-ground (aerial) parts of hemp plants but is concentrated in the fine, hair-like, resinous glands (trichomes) which produce a shiny, sticky, secretion resembling crystals or frosting. These protuberances develop along the outer surface of the leaves, bracts (leaf-like structures around the flowers) and stems as soon as the plant starts to produce buds.

Trichomes secrete and store phytocannabinoids and essential oils as part of the plant's natural defence mechanisms. Their bitter taste, strong aroma and antimicrobial properties deter fungi, insects and animals and provide some protection against harmful UV rays. This means that the leaves at the top of the plant have the highest phytocannabinoid content.

The quantity of CBD obtained from each plant depends not only on the method of extraction but also on its growing conditions, the time of harvest, whether the flowers or just the leaves and/or stems are used and how the plant matter is stored immediately after harvest. CBD levels tend to reduce as the plant matures, so selecting the right time for harvesting and processing is a balancing act.

When CBD can be legally extracted from low THC hemp flowers (such as in the US and Canada, but not within the EU), the maximum concentration is obtained by separating the flower heads from the leaves and stems for processing. The resulting extract usually contains more than 10% CBD. When legislation dictates that CBD can only be taken from the stems of hemp plants, as in the UK, the resulting extract usually contains between 3 and 5% CBD.

There are several ways to extract CBD from hemp plants, of which the gold-standard method uses liquid carbon dioxide (CO_2) as a solvent. When buying a CBD product, look for those that are produced by 'supercritical CO_2 extraction' (sometimes just described as CO_2 extraction) if you want the best quality (this is usually proudly mentioned on the manufacturer's website and on the label). This method uses liquid CO_2 at a controlled pressure and temperature to separate the oil from the plant material and dissolve out the cannabinoids and essential oils.

This process produces the purest extract without contaminants such as heavy metals or pesticides. It also removes most of the chlorophyll, which, while not bad for you, can give a bitter flavour. Crucially, the carbon dioxide evaporates away from the final extract without leaving behind any traces of solvent.

CO_2 extraction separates out as much as 92% of the cannabinoids present. The downside is that it is an expensive form of processing hemp for CBD so the final products cost more to buy, reflecting their quality.

Supercritical CO_2 extraction is also used to decaffeinate coffee and to extract pure essential oils used in high-end perfumery.

CBD can also be obtained by soaking hemp material in a solvent, such as a hydrocarbon (e.g. propane), to dissolve out the cannabinoids. The resulting solution is then distilled and evaporated to remove the solvent and recover the phytocannabinoid extract. There have been health concerns about using hydrocarbons for extraction, as any solvent residues remaining in the extract are potentially toxic. I recommend that you avoid these by only selecting products that say they are produced by CO_2 extraction. Some manufacturers use natural solvents such as olive oil or alcohol (ethanol) to avoid leaving a toxic residue. The resulting extracts have lower concentrations of CBD, however, and include chlorophyll which taints the taste.

Purification of CBD oil

Whichever extraction method is used, the resulting extracts are rather murky-looking – some on the market taste really rank. Look for products that have undergone additional filtering – some are almost transparent and described as 'filter-clear' – to remove unwanted plant matter such as lipids, waxes and, in the case of natural solvents, chlorophyll. This produces a clearer liquid with a less earthy or bitter taste.

Extracts may also undergo an additional decarboxylation process, in which any remaining acidic cannabidiolic acid (CBDA) is converted to the beneficial, active CBD. Products that still contain some inactive CBDA are sometimes described as 'raw' and are less effective.

Depending on the purification methods used, manufacturers can produce a:

- Full-spectrum CBD oil (containing all the phyto-cannabinoids present in hemp plants, including low levels of THC)
- Broad-spectrum CBD extract (containing all the phyto-cannabinoids except THC, which is removed)
- Narrow-spectrum product (sometimes called isolate) in which the only phytocannabinoid present is CBD

(See 'What the terms mean' on page 102 for more on the different types of CBD products available to buy.)

Once the desired CBD-rich extract is obtained, it is dissolved in a carrier oil such as olive oil, hemp seed oil or coconut oil and this final product is known as CBD oil. Diluting CBD extract with a carrier oil allows manufacturers to produce a standardised product that contains a known concentration of CBD and also increases the amount of CBD we absorb. Essential oils such as lemon, orange or peppermint are sometimes added to provide a more pleasant flavour when consumed as drops. Alternatively, the CBD oil can be made into CBD capsules.

To produce gummies, the CBD extract is combined with fruit juice, corn syrup and natural flavourings to produce a flavoured, edible pastille or chew.

When making a CBD vape, the CBD extract is dissolved in vegetable glycerine and propylene glycol so that it becomes suitable for inhalation.

For topical salves, the CBD is dissolved in carriers such as shea butter, aloe vera and beeswax and scented with aromatherapy essential oils to create a balm.

These different ways of using CBD provide lots of choices, so you can select a product based on your personal preference. Some people, like myself, prefer capsules because they do not like the earthy flavour of hemp extracts. Others prefer the more rapid effects of using CBD oil drops and holding them in the mouth for a couple of minutes for absorption through the lining of the mouth. CBD ointments and creams can also be used in addition to an oral supplement to provide local relief for muscle, joint or other types of pain.

5

How to Use CBD Safely

Thanks to the increasing interest in the potential benefits of CBD, there are many different CBD products on the market, and more are appearing all the time. While CBD-infused drinks and foods are mainly used for recreational purposes, they can provide a significant dose – some beverages contain as much as 25mg CBD per can. People who want to treat specific symptoms usually choose more medicinal formats such as drops, sprays or capsules, as these are easier to take in higher doses without the calories supplied by drinks and snacks. Whichever form of CBD you use, it is important to be aware of the following safety considerations.

In 2018, the journal *Medical Cannabis and Cannabinoids* published a review entitled 'The Trouble with CBD Oil', which highlighted a number of concerns about the quality and safety of some CBD products in the Netherlands and elsewhere in the world. Many of the new products entering the market are virtually unchecked due to a lack of regulatory control. Some are produced by amateurs for family and friends and have unknown content and quality. Those that are produced using solvent extraction (see page 93) may contain harmful solvents, while others are contaminated with pesticides, metal particles, heavy metals, moulds, bacteria or fungal poisons. A surprising number have incorrect or misleading labels and contain more (or in some cases less) CBD than claimed. Others have unlabelled or unknown amounts of THC, or even synthetic cannabinoids (see page 46) which could produce unwanted 'psychoactive' side effects similar to those associated with marijuana. A worrying number also make illegal claims, such as preventing or treating certain diseases, in order to encourage sales – such claims can only be made by licensed, medical drugs, and only when authorised. Another problem is that CBD products sold as supplements may recommend excessively high doses (above 70mg per day), which are best used only under medical supervision.

Although the report raised concerns about risks, it did acknowledge the potential of CBD to become an effective treatment for a growing number of health problems. However, because CBD is often used by severely ill people, it is now blurring the line between what is a food supplement and what is a medicine. An important difference between the two is that medicines are considered *unsafe* until their safety is proven in clinical trials, while the safety of supplements is assumed (even taken for granted) until proven otherwise.

Luckily, though, as the World Health Organization concluded in their 2018 report, pure CBD causes few side effects, isn't addictive and is unlikely to pose a danger to the public – for example, through causing dangerous driving or intoxication, as with alcohol.[1] You are unlikely to be able to 'overdose' if you take a product containing more CBD than advertised on the label (although this is not advisable). But still, safety concerns have been raised about products that are widely available in the UK and elsewhere – even those bought in shops on the high street, not just those obtained online from dubious sources.

In 2017, for example, a study published in the *Journal of the American Medical Association* tested eighty-four CBD extracts bought over the internet.[2] Of these, thirty-six contained less CBD than claimed (making them less effective) and twenty-two contained more CBD than claimed which, while making them good value, meant that users were taking higher doses than they realised. This could lead to consumers exceeding recommended upper doses for use as supplements. Only twenty-six of the eighty-four products were accurately labelled for their CBD content. THC was detected in more than a fifth of samples, with some products containing levels sufficient to produce intoxication or mental impairment. CBDA was found in thirteen samples, suggesting that the products were not professionally processed according to good quality standards. The products most frequently mis-labelled were CBD vapes (in 87.5% of cases).

Unfortunately, things are little better in the UK. In June 2019, the Centre for Medicinal Cannabis published an audit of thirty CBD oils available on high streets and websites.[3] Around two out of three products tested contained less than 90% of the level of CBD claimed on the label, which not only makes them poor value for money but means they will not deliver the benefits expected at a particular dose. One CBD product contained no detectable cannabinoids at all despite an eye-watering price tag of £90 per pack. Anyone using this product would, understandably, assume that the benefits of CBD are all based on hype as they would experience no discernible effects.

When it comes to safety, more than half the products tested contained excessive amounts of the legally controlled cannabinoid THC. Not only does this make the products illegal (if they contain more than 1mg THC per pack), but it could also lead to unexpected drowsiness, mental impairment or 'stoned' side effects. In addition, seven products contained cannabinol (CBN), which is formed from the breakdown of THC and is also a legally controlled drug.

Another safety issue was that eight samples contained levels of certain solvents (dichloromethane or cyclohexane) that exceeded those allowed by food regulations. These solvents are potentially toxic and could lead to side effects such as nausea or diarrhoea. These solvent traces were also inconsistent with the advertised method of CO_2 extraction – meaning the manufacturers were using cheap extraction methods instead of the more expensive, quality process they claimed. Four samples did not even feature a batch number or use-by date. Without a use-by date, products could be sold that were past their prime (for example, with rancid tastes due to deterioration of their oils) and, without a batch number, it would not be easy to recall the products if serious safety issues were identified.

These findings underline the importance of checking the quality of the CBD products you buy to ensure you get the dose of CBD you expect (and are paying for) without unwanted contaminants. Fortunately, this is possible as long as you select products that are made to a pharmaceutical standard known as current good manufacturing practice (GMP or CGMP).

What is GMP?

Current good manufacturing practice refers to the rules and regulations that ensure the consistent quality of medical drugs, which can also be applied to the manufacture of quality supplements such as CBD oil. This quality standard ensures that labelled claims are accurate, with each liquid extract or capsule containing only the ingredients listed, in the amounts specified, with no contaminants.

The principles of GMP ensure, for example, that premises are of a high standard and inspected regularly, there are appropriate levels of hygiene to prevent contamination and that every stage of the process is documented and double-checked. Samples of all raw materials are analysed to confirm their identity and purity, all ingredients are properly prepared and weighed, and finished supplements are tested to ensure they contain the labelled amounts of CBD and only trace amounts of THC. Samples of all raw ingredients and finished products are also retained and stored for future reference, and records ensure that each batch can be traced back from product to field. Studies are also carried out to confirm the stability and 'shelf life' of finished products.

In the UK, compliance with GMP regulations is assessed by the Medicines and Healthcare products Regulatory Agency (MHRA). In the US, the Food and Drug Administration (FDA) oversees compliance with regulations relating to the

Dietary Supplement Current Good Manufacturing Practices (CGMPs) for quality control.

Not all manufacturers making CBD supplements comply with GMP guidelines because of the extra cost and effort involved. I strongly urge you to check that the CBD supplements you buy *are* produced in GMP accredited facilities. To do this, check the manufacturer's website (they should proudly mention this in their 'About Us' page), or use your browser to search for the manufacturer's name plus the term 'GMP'. If you can't find any mention of GMP associated with the manufacturer, I advise that you move on to a different brand.

Good quality products sold online are both made to GMP standards and will have an independent batch certificate of testing that confirms the level of CBD and that only low, trace levels of THC (e.g. less than 0.05%) are present. Look for a clickable link to the batch certificate next to your chosen product on the website.

Alternatively, buy your CBD products from an accredited national pharmacy chain rather than a health food shop. Following the recognition that some CBD products on sale on UK high streets had inaccurate labelling, big pharmacy chains now require manufacturers to supply certification from independent tests to prove their products are legal and of acceptable quality.

In the UK, any CBD product that contains more than 1mg of THC within the pack as a whole (rather than per dose) is currently illegal.

Manufacturers who are genuinely concerned about quality and safety are banding together to form trade associations that set their own compliance standards in an attempt to stamp out poor quality products. In the UK, for example, the Centre for Medicinal Cannabis has drawn up a Cannabinoid Industry Quality Charter made up of seven pillars of regulations, relating to testing, labelling, manufacturing, undetectable amounts of controlled substances, marketing ethics, sustainability and social impact.

What the terms mean

Different CBD products provide a different blend of cannabinoids and you will usually find that products are described on the pack as having a full spectrum, broad spectrum or narrow spectrum. These terms reflect whether CBD is present on its own, or with all or just some of the additional cannabinoids that normally occur alongside it within the plant.

Full-spectrum extracts contain CBD plus all the cannabinoids naturally present within hemp plants. This will include trace amounts of THC at levels that should be too low to have a psychoactive effect (in other words, they should not produce a 'high'). These supplements are often considered superior as they provide a full entourage effect (meaning the cannabinoids act together to provide greater than expected benefits – see page 23).

Broad-spectrum extracts contain CBD plus most of the other natural cannabinoids, but have had all their THC content removed. These supplements are ideal for those who want to take CBD but do not want to risk ingesting any THC (for example, if you are subjected to drug testing at work).

Narrow-spectrum extracts, also known as **CBD isolates**, contain high levels of just one cannabinoid – CBD – with levels of other cannabinoids greatly reduced or absent. CBD isolates may be extracted from hemp plants or produced synthetically in a laboratory. As the legislation currently stands in the EU, CBD isolates are illegal in food supplements, although they can be used in vapes. The status of highly purified CBD products from which the other cannabinoids have been selectively removed by filtration is less clear. Some manufacturers are avoiding them until the EU has completed its novel foods safety assessment of hemp extracts and their position is more certain (see pages 12–15).

What the numbers mean

Some CBD products may list on their label the amount of CBD they contain in milligrams (e.g. 10mg or 15mg) while others will list a percentage (e.g. 5% or 10%).

In some countries, such as the UK, the total amount of CBD present within the whole package is also listed (e.g. 250mg CBD in a 10ml bottle of CBD oil, or 900mg CBD in a whole pack of sixty CBD capsules, each of which therefore provides 15mg CBD).

There are several reasons for the different systems.

CBD oil labels tend to use percentages as it's difficult to know exactly how big a drop your pipette might deliver. The percentage refers to the concentration of CBD within the product. So, if a product is described as having a strength of 5%, then CBD makes up 5% of the total product and the other listed ingredients (e.g. hemp seed oil) will account for the remaining 95%.

If a 10ml bottle of CBD oil contains 200mg CBD, then every single millilitre should contain 20mg CBD (200mg divided by 10ml). A drop delivered from the pipette is usually around one-twentieth of a millilitre, or 0.05ml. So, if a single millilitre of oil contains 20mg CBD, it will provide around 1mg CBD per single drop.

What is the best CBD dose?

All products should have clear recommendations on daily dose. How much CBD you take will vary depending on the strength of the product and the reason you are taking it. Some people may use CBD regularly, every day, or even several times a day, while others may only use it when they feel in need of relaxation, when they experience a pain flare-up or at times when they have difficulty falling asleep. Always follow the manufacturer's guidance on the dose and frequency of use of their product as this is based on the CBD concentration present. Do not exceed the manufacturer's recommended dose except under medical advice and supervision.

It's best to start at a low dose and slowly increase (for example, on a weekly basis) to find what works best for you. Around one in ten people appear to metabolise CBD slowly, which means they only need a low dose to notice an effect.

A typical CBD starting dose when using it as a food supplement, for whatever reason, is 6mg to 10mg CBD taken one to three times per day, or 15mg taken once or twice a day. When prescribed as a medicine (for example, to treat some rare forms of epilepsy), however, higher starting doses are used.

Food Supplements

CBD is classed as a food supplement for legal purposes and this term must appear on the label. Food supplements are concentrated sources of vitamins, minerals or other substances (such as CBD) which are derived from foods. They are usually taken in small, measured doses for their nutritional or other effects on the body. Food supplements are regulated under food law and are only allowed to make claims that appear on the EU Register of Nutrition and Health Claims. There are no authorised health claims for CBD so manufacturers are not allowed to say what CBD is used for.

High doses of CBD are best treated as a medicine and only used under medical supervision (for example, if your doctor agrees to support your use of CBD to treat anxiety, pain or other symptoms). This is partly to monitor its safe use, and partly because people who need higher doses are likely to have physical or emotional problems that merit ongoing medical care.

In the UK, the Cannabis Trades Association recommends that, as a food supplement, CBD should not be used at doses above 200mg per day, until there is clarification from the Medicines and Healthcare products Regulatory Agency (MHRA).

The European Industrial Hemp Association have proposed an even lower cut-off for food supplements, so that members should not recommend more than a maximum daily intake of 160mg CBD for the average adult.

As a doctor, I feel more comfortable suggesting that you should not take more than 70mg cannabidiol (CBD) per day, in total, without talking to your own GP first.

If you have any medical condition or are taking any prescribed drugs, always speak to your doctor before using CBD (or unlicensed medical marijuana) and check for interactions with your medication. If taking an over-the-counter medicine, ask your pharmacist's advice. If they are unable to help, there is a useful drugs interaction checker which includes cannabidiol at Drugs.com.

Which form of CBD is best for you?

CBD extracts are available in the form of gummies, drops, oral sprays, capsules, vapes, melts and topical balms. Recently, the popularity of foods and drinks infused with CBD has also skyrocketed.

In the US, for example, a 2019 Consumer Reports survey found the most popular way to use CBD was in these 'edibles' (35%), although many people also used other types of CBD products including CBD drops or sprays (30%), vaping devices (30%) and topical rubs or creams (21%). Only 16% preferred cigarettes or smokable forms of CBD, and just 15% took CBD in pill or capsule form.

New CBD products are launched almost daily and a wide range of CBD-infused products is now available, such as water, fruit juice, beers, chocolates, marshmallows and even intimate lubricants.

Selecting a CBD product depends on personal choice and the reason why you are taking it. Most people are used to swallowing medicines in the form of capsules or tablets rather than as drops or tinctures, which are generally seen as old-fashioned or, at best, artisanal. Most CBD oils look dark and murky and have an earthy taste, even when disguised with flavourings. A few CBD oils are more highly filtered and distilled to look clearer and these are more palatable – especially if you are holding the drops under your tongue for two minutes to maximise absorption. These are the products to go for if you want a CBD oil in a dropper bottle but dislike the taste of hemp.

As a medic, I prefer capsules. These have a more conventional, therapeutic feel as well as the advantage of no unpleasant taste. They also provide an exact dose (when made to GMP standards) rather than the guesswork of using a dropper and counting drops.

Gummies are increasingly popular and can taste delicious, so you will need good self-control not to keep taking them in the same way you might eat a pack of sweets!

CBD can also be absorbed through the skin via patches, salves, creams and balms. The CBD in these products interacts with local receptors in skin cells, skin nerve fibres and skin glands. Some is also absorbed into the body to produce more widespread effects. If you have a skin condition, or a single painful joint, rubbing in a CBD balm can complement the effects of a CBD supplement taken orally.

When selecting a CBD product, check it is made to GMP standards and decide whether you want a narrow-spectrum product (supplying mostly pure CBD), a broad-spectrum product (with no THC) or a full-spectrum product for a full entourage effect (see page 94). You will also need to decide if you want a product that states it is organic or made in a fully sustainable way, if these considerations are important to you.

CBD infused sportswear is available in the US.[5] The manufacturer states that microscopic droplets of CBD are wrapped in a protective polymer coating to form microcapsules that are embedded into the fibre panels using a patented textile finishing treatment. Friction between the fabric and your skin during a workout causes the microcapsules to open and gradually release CBD, which is claimed to reduce pain and inflammation after a workout (such as delayed-onset muscle soreness which typically comes on twelve to twenty-four hours after a vigorous exercise session). It's possible this might work but applying a CBD balm or taking a CBD supplement is likely to be more effective!

How quickly does CBD work?

The speed at which CBD starts to have an effect will depend on the delivery method you choose. A CBD oil or spray held under the tongue is absorbed more quickly into the bloodstream than capsules taken by mouth, so you may notice a relaxing effect within just a few minutes, and this can last for up to twelve hours, depending on the dose.

Taking CBD orally

When taking CBD orally, for example, via gummies or capsules, some CBD is broken down by stomach acid but 95% of the dose successfully crosses the intestinal wall into the bloodstream. However, the absorbed CBD is then transported straight to your liver where significant amounts are broken down by enzymes. As a result, only 13 to 19% of the CBD dose 'survives' to reach the rest of your body – so you need a higher dose than when absorbing CBD straight into the bloodstream by holding it under your tongue (as described below). This also means there is a delay of thirty to ninety minutes after swallowing a dose before noticeable effects occur. The maximum effect usually occurs two to three hours after swallowing CBD, with effects lasting for around three to five hours, and up to twelve hours, depending on the dose.

Because CBD dissolves in fat rather than water, it is a good idea to take your CBD with a high-fat meal if you are taking it orally as this boosts absorption by as much as five times. When taking prescribed CBD, follow your doctor's instructions on whether or not to take it with food. You will usually be advised to take it consistently either on an empty stomach or after a meal, but don't chop and change or blood levels will fluctuate (increasing the risk of side effects if they rise too high, or of becoming ineffective if levels fall too low).

Taking CBD under the tongue

When CBD is taken via a sublingual spray or drops, which are held under the tongue for two minutes, it is absorbed directly through the lining of the mouth into the bloodstream (although some will inevitably be swallowed). As a result, two or three times more (up to 35%) will reach the bloodstream compared with swallowing the whole dose, and most people will notice an effect within twenty minutes or so. The effect will tend to last longer, too, for an average of five to twelve hours, depending on the dose.

Inhaling CBD

When using a vape, the amount of CBD that reaches the bloodstream via the lungs ranges from 11 to 45% of the dose, depending on how deeply you inhale and for how long you hold your breath before breathing out. The maximum effect usually occurs within fifteen to thirty minutes and then tapers off over two to three hours. See safety concerns over vaping CBD and other cannabis products, page 117.

Intravaginal CBD Products

CBD products prescribed as vaginal pessaries (for example, to help menstrual cramps or endometriosis) and as rectal suppositories (e.g. to treat prostate pain) are absorbed across a mucous membrane and the amount that enters the bloodstream is similar to that seen with drops absorbed under the tongue.

Do not use CBD-infused tampons and never add CBD drops to a tampon yourself, as is irresponsibly recommended in some forums. It is unknown how a CBD tampon will affect the risk of toxic shock syndrome (TSS).

TSS is a rare but serious illness caused by bacteria (*Staphylococcus aureus*) which live in or on the body, including the vagina. Under certain circumstances, some strains of these bacteria start to make a toxin called TSST-1. Why they do this is unknown, but it has been related to the use of high-absorbency tampons. TSS can also occur if a wound such as a burn or insect bite becomes infected with the bacteria that make this toxin.

While most people develop antibodies against the toxin and become naturally immune, some do not. Symptoms of TSS include a high fever, vomiting, diarrhoea, muscle aches, rash, dizziness (low blood pressure), severe flu-like feelings and confusion. It is treated easily in the early stages but will quickly become serious if it is left and can prove fatal.

How often should you take CBD?

When taken orally, CBD stays in your bloodstream for several days, but as levels fall the benefits wear off until they become unnoticeable. The effects of CBD supplements (at doses that are usually less than 70mg) typically last for around three to five hours. When taken for stress and to aid relaxation, manufacturers usually recommend taking CBD twice a day.

Taking CBD regularly, two or three times a day, will help to maintain even blood levels of CBD, giving you better results than when taking a higher dose just once a day. Don't be tempted to take all of a day's dose in one go or you are more likely to experience potential side effects (such as drowsiness), and the benefits will wear off more quickly than when taking the same amount but divided into two or three doses spread throughout the day.

However, if you are taking CBD to improve your sleep, you only need to take it at night, usually around twenty to thirty minutes before bedtime. Oral sprays and drops held in the mouth tend to work more quickly than capsules that are swallowed (see above), so the exact timing will depend on the formulation and dose.

If you are taking CBD oil for anxiety or pain and want to reduce the chance of symptoms reappearing as the dose wears off, you may find it helpful to take the supplement at regular intervals, such as three times a day, for continuous benefits. Don't exceed the manufacturer's stated dose except under medical advice, however.

You will find more detailed advice for using CBD for specific conditions in the chapters that follow.

Do not use CBD while pregnant or breastfeeding

CBD (and THC and other cannabinoids) readily cross the placenta to reach the developing baby and are also excreted into breast milk. Research into the development of the central nervous system suggests that exposure to cannabinoids in the womb may lead to subtle changes that could, possibly, affect the baby's future personality and emotional wellbeing, although this is not yet established.[6]

Will CBD show up during drug testing?

A CBD oil that is made to pharmaceutical standards (GMP) and which has been independently tested and certified to contain no detectable THC (or CBN, which is a breakdown product of THC and is also a controlled drug) should not represent a risk in drug testing. This is because tests that determine the likelihood of marijuana use only detect controlled substances such as THC (and CBN). If you have to take part in drug testing (e.g. in elite sports), always check with the relevant authorities whether or not you are allowed to use CBD (cannabidiol) according to your particular circumstances.

At the time of writing, according to the World Anti-Doping Agency (WADA), which regulates drug policies for sports organisations across the world, all natural and synthetic cannabinoids are banned except for cannabidiol (CBD).[7] However, they add that athletes should be aware that some CBD oils and tinctures extracted from cannabis plants may also contain THC and other cannabinoids that could result in a positive test for a prohibited cannabinoid.

Regulations are in a state of flux and may change at any time, so always check. It's also important to know that hemp seed oil products can also contain unexpected levels of THC (see chapter eight). For these reasons, many athletes are turning to a natural cannabinoid-like molecule known as PEA for relaxation and pain relief (see chapter nine).

Side effects of CBD

Most people do not experience side effects when taking food supplement doses of CBD (typically less than 70mg per day), but everyone is different and will respond in different ways.

In an online survey of 2,409 people taking CBD, only minor side effects were reported, of which the most common overall were dry mouth when used as an oral spray or drops (11.1%), euphoria (6.4%), hunger (6.4%), red eyes (2.7%) and feeling sleepy (1.8%).[8] There is no certainty about the quality of CBD products used by those taking part in the survey, however, and some may have contained unlabelled amounts of THC or other substances that produced these effects – for example, euphoria and hunger are more usually associated with THC than with CBD. Even so, no serious side effects were noted.

Other side effects that have occasionally been reported when taking CBD include lack of dream recall or vivid dreams, insomnia, agitation, chills, fever, loss of appetite or a skin rash.

If you experience what you think may be a side effect of CBD, then stop taking it to see whether or not the unwanted adverse effects disappear. If they do, then, depending on their severity, you may wish to start taking CBD again to see if the unwanted symptoms recur. If they do recur, they are likely to reflect how you, as an individual, respond to CBD. If you are concerned in any way, then see your doctor.

Avoid CBD if you are taking any medications with which it is known to interact.

Only adults over the age of eighteen should use CBD supplements – under this age it should only be taken if medically advised.

Studies into the safety of high doses of CBD

Researchers have tested the safety and tolerability of high doses of CBD in healthy volunteers. The amounts used varied from 1,500mg to 6,000mg CBD as single doses, and 750mg to 1,500mg CBD as multiple doses taken twice a day for six days. The effects of these high doses were then compared with an inactive placebo (a dummy oil containing no CBD).[9]

Despite these very high doses, CBD was generally well tolerated. The most commonly reported side effects were diarrhoea, nausea, headache and drowsiness. All side effects were classed as mild or moderate, with none classed as severe or serious.

This study found that, when CBD was taken with a high-fat meal, its absorption and blood levels increased 4.85 times more than when taken on an empty stomach. This could be a good thing to obtain the best results, but also suggests that you should take a lower dose of CBD if taking it with fatty foods. It also suggests that you should take a CBD supplement consistently, either with or without food, to obtain the same effects. The results also confirmed that taking CBD twice a day helped to maintain blood levels to get beneficial effects throughout the day.

It is important to note that the very high doses of CBD used in this study were for research purposes only. I recommend that you do not take more than 70mg CBD per day without talking to your doctor. If you have symptoms that need a higher dose, you most likely need additional medical support.

Taking CBD with other medicines

If you are taking any prescribed or over-the-counter drugs or other herbal medicines, it is important to check with your doctor before taking CBD and to find out whether or not there are any known interactions. CBD affects the action of intestinal and liver enzymes that break down many prescribed medicines. If CBD *slows down* the breakdown of your medicine, then blood levels of the drug will stay higher for longer, which could lead to serious side effects. If CBD *speeds up* the breakdown of your medicine, then its levels in your blood will fall more quickly so your medication becomes less effective.

If the patient information leaflet that comes with your medication says to avoid grapefruit juice, then do not take CBD. Grapefruit juice affects the enzymes that break down certain medicines in a similar way. If the leaflet does not mention grapefruit juice it is still advisable to check with your doctor before taking CBD.

Safety concerns over vaping

For smokers who are addicted to nicotine, the relative risk of vaping (using a personal battery-powered vaporiser) is considered less harmful than inhaling the fumes from burning tobacco. Less harmful does not mean safe, however, and vaping is definitely not as safe as inhaling fresh air. The same risk reduction does not apply with non-addictive substances such as CBD, which can easily be taken by mouth rather than having to be inhaled. There is also growing evidence that vaping in itself can damage the lungs – whether or not it contains active ingredients such as CBD.

CBD e-liquids designed for vaping contain a concentrated CBD extract plus propylene glycol, vegetable glycerine (glycerol) and, usually, a flavouring agent.

In February 2018, the US Army Public Health Center issued a public health alert after ninety-three soldiers and marines experienced serious medical problems that were considered possible side effects from vaping synthetic cannabinoid products. The symptoms reported included palpitations, headaches, vomiting, disorientation, dizziness, agitation and seizures, which led to the hospitalisation of sixty soldiers and, sadly, there were two deaths.[10]

Most recently, in October 2019, in the USA, the FDA issued a warning for people to stop using vape products containing THC and any vaping products obtained off the street or from other illicit sources, following over 1,000 reports of suspected associated lung injuries, including some deaths. While the exact cause of these lung problems remains uncertain, there appears to be a link with fatty additives such as vitamin E acetate and triglycerides which may irritate the airways.

Some of these health issues may also relate to poor quality products and the presence of contaminants. For example, a study published in January 2019 revealed that five out of nine commercially available CBD vape products contained harmful contaminants – four even contained an illegal synthetic cannabinoid that has psychoactive effects. Another contained a drug that is used orally to suppress coughs, but which has no beneficial effects when inhaled into the lungs (and could well be harmful).[11]

Another safety concern is that the quantity of CBD present in vape liquids is often higher than stated on the label. For example, scientists who analysed two commercially available e-liquids found that both contained more than twice the amount of CBD stated on the packs.[12]

Even without contaminants, there is increasing concern that vape additives used to thin the liquid and keep it moist can create harmful chemicals (such as acetaldehyde and formaldehyde) when converted to vapour at high temperatures. These chemicals are known to damage the lungs and blood vessels and some may increase the risk of cancer. Unfortunately, newer designs of e-cigarette and vape devices generate more of these damaging chemicals than older devices because their battery power is higher, creating higher temperatures.[14]

Another concern is that vaping aerosols contain metal particles which originate from the metallic coil used to heat e-liquids, and from solders and wicks. When inhaled, these tiny particles lodge in the lungs and damage the airways to trigger inflammation and reduce immune defences. It's now thought that vaping may increase the risk of lung infections, chronic obstructive pulmonary disease (COPD) as well as lung cancers.

Other reports suggest vaping can raise blood pressure and increase the risk of a heart attack. CBD undoubtedly offers many health benefits when taken in the much safer form of drops, gummies, capsules or sprays. There is no reason to neutralise these benefits by inhaling CBD e-liquids. Having said that, some prescribed forms of medical marijuana are dispensed as vapes as treatments for conditions, in cases where the benefits are deemed to outweigh the risks.

I don't advise using CBD in vape form (or any other e-liquid, including medical marijuana) unless specifically prescribed by your doctor after a careful assessment of risks versus benefits.

CBD is a useful supplement when used wisely, at sensible doses. The best way to use CBD is via oral or capsules or drops, and as CBD-infused balms. If you are receiving medical treatment, talk to your doctor before taking it and check for interactions with any medicines you are taking.

6

CBD for Pain and Other Physical Conditions

CBD is increasingly being used for a wide range of physical ailments and conditions. Some of these uses are supported by research, while others are based on anecdote and personal experience. Even where there is good evidence to support the use of CBD for conditions such as pain, products that are sold as supplements cannot make unauthorised health claims, so manufacturers can't tell you why people use their products – even for general purposes such as relaxation. They certainly aren't able to make medicinal claims for effects such as pain relief – this would position their products as medicines, which requires licensing and evidence of safety and effectiveness from extensive (and expensive) clinical trials.

In general, CBD is CBD and provides the same benefits in whatever form you take it. Salves are best for skin conditions as it is delivered directly to where it is needed; otherwise, you can use a spray, drops or capsules depending on which you prefer.

Within the UK, there are two main groups of supplements – those classed as food supplements, which are regulated by the Food Standards Agency under food laws, and those licensed as traditional herbal medicines, which are overseen by the Medicines and Healthcare products Regulatory Agency (MHRA).

Food supplements contain concentrated substances extracted from food sources, which are taken in small, measured doses for their nutritional or other effects on the body. These food supplements are allowed to make specific, authorised statements relating to health benefits only if they are listed in the EU Register of Nutrition and Health Claims. These statements mainly relate to vitamins, minerals, essential fatty acids (such as fish oils) and certain extracts such as plant sterols (which are used to lower cholesterol).

Herbal medicines are licensed by the MHRA to treat a range of 'minor' conditions that are appropriate for self-treatment, such as stress (*Rhodiola rosea*), the common cold (*Pelargonium sidoides*), low mood and mild anxiety (St John's wort) or sleep disturbances (valerian). While these licensed herbal medicines undergo quality assurance testing and safety assessments in the same way as conventional pharmaceutical drugs, they don't have to prove their effectiveness for treating these conditions – their licences are based on a long history of traditional use (which presupposes they are effective or people would have stopped using them centuries ago). These herbal medicines have the advantage of being able to say on the pack what conditions they are used for (but can still only use authorised statements). They also include a patient information leaflet that details possible side effects, drug interactions and who should not take them – just like with medical drugs.

Other herbs that have traditional therapeutic uses but which are also used in the kitchen are classed as food supplements rather than as herbal medicines. Examples include globe artichoke, sage, garlic, turmeric and Korean ginseng. As food supplements, they can't make any unauthorised health claims or mention on their label what they are used for unless a claim has been authorised by the European Food Safety Authority (EFSA).

CBD falls into this latter group. As there are currently no EU authorised health claims for CBD and it is not licensed as a traditional herbal medicine, it can only be sold in the UK if it doesn't make any health or medical claims. This is why there is no information on CBD packs to indicate what it is used for. It means you have to do your own online research and read articles in newspapers and magazines, or self-help books such as this one, to find out how CBD might help you.

While many people – myself included – take CBD as a well-being supplement to aid relaxation and promote sleep, many people rely on CBD to help them cope with long-term painful conditions and/or to reduce anxiety and mood swings.

As scientists have unravelled the complexities of the body's own endocannabinoid system, it has become clear that changes in how this system regulates interactions between our cells – especially nerve and immune cells – underpin almost every type of human disease. Intriguingly, there is growing evidence that some long-term physical and mental health conditions may be related to producing fewer endocannabinoids than we need to maintain good health. This is where CBD fits in, by helping to boost our endocannabinoid system and restoring balance.

In this chapter we will look at the physical conditions that CBD is most commonly used to treat, and we will look at the research – or lack of it – to support its effectiveness.

If you have a medical condition, always talk to your doctor before taking CBD or any supplement. It's also important to check for potential interactions with any medication you are taking.

CBD and pain-related conditions

Pain is the most common reason for seeking healthcare advice and is the underlying reason for over half of all medical consultations. It is also the most common reason for taking CBD.

It is estimated that, worldwide, one in five adults are living with pain at any one time, which may be acute (sudden onset), intermittent (comes and goes) or persistent (constant and unrelenting). Once pain lasts longer than a certain period of time (usually considered to be either three months or six months, depending on the definition used) it is described as chronic or long-term pain.

As many as one in ten adults are newly diagnosed with chronic pain every year. The most common causes are osteoarthritis, rheumatoid arthritis, operations, injuries, back problems and cancer. Other causes of persistent pain include neuralgia (nerve pain), fibromyalgia (widespread soft tissue pain), muscle pain, multiple sclerosis, irritable bowel syndrome and other conditions affecting the gut such as gallbladder disease and diverticulitis.

The Burden of Pain

According to the *British Medical Journal*, an astonishing 43.5% of adults in the UK are living with chronic pain (in this case defined as lasting at least three months) – in other words, just under 28 million people. This increases with age, from 14.3% among those aged eighteen to twenty-five, to 62% of over-seventy-fives.[1]

Not surprisingly, living with pain has a significant impact on your quality of life. No matter where the pain is, its frequency or severity, pain reduces your ability to carry out day-to-day activities and do the things you enjoy. Joint pain can affect your ability to move around and go out, for example, so you don't feel like socialising. Pain can also make it difficult to concentrate on other things and, if it interrupts your sleep, can lead to increasing tiredness and irritability.

What causes pain?

Pain is an unpleasant sensation triggered when special nerve endings (nociceptors), which are present in most parts of the body, are stimulated. Once a pain receptor is activated, it sends nerve messages along the nerve fibre to the spinal cord which relays them up to the brain, where pain is perceived.

Some nerve endings are very sensitive and give a warning to alert you to potential damage from firm pressure (e.g. a tight shoe), unusual stretching (such as bending a finger backwards) or a change in temperature. Others are less sensitive and are only activated by severe stimulation, such as when we cut, prick or burn ourselves.

Pain is subjective and how severe it is does not always correspond to any obvious signs of disease or damage. It can vary from a mild ache – for example, due to a slight muscle strain – to an unbearable and excruciating pain such as that experienced from kidney stones. There are many types of pain in between – for example, the pain you experience when you sprain a ligament or have a toothache.

Not all types of pain are due to illness or injury, however. The stresses and strains of everyday life, and even normal body functions, can lead to a degree of pain, such as tension headache and period pains.

Pain can be deep or superficial and may be described as: aching, gnawing, dragging, throbbing, stabbing, burning, stinging, bruising, sharp, dull, crushing, tight, constant or colicky (comes and goes in waves).

Although pain is an unpleasant experience, it is designed to let you know when something is wrong. Many illnesses, even minor ones such as a common cold, cause aches and pains to ensure you rest while your body fights the infection and heals. Once you are aware you have a problem, however, the pain has served its purpose and you can take steps to treat it using painkilling drugs.

The problem with analgesic drugs

One of the main reasons why people decide to try CBD for pain relief is that standard analgesics such as aspirin, paracetamol/acetaminophen, non-steroidal anti-inflammatory drugs (NSAIDs such as ibuprofen) and even opiates such as codeine are not that effective. Common variations in our genes mean that not all of the conventional painkillers work for everyone.

Paracetamol is believed to work through a direct effect on the brain to reduce pain and lower a fever. It has little, if any, effects against inflammation and is often unhelpful in conditions where there is swelling or stiffness. For example, studies suggest that paracetamol is not that effective for reducing back pain or the pain associated with osteoarthritis of the hip or knee.

Non-steroidal anti-inflammatory drugs (NSAIDs) such as aspirin and ibuprofen have a painkilling action that is comparable to that of paracetamol when taken in a single dose. It's only when taken regularly that they have lasting effects against pain and inflammation – it takes up to a week of regular use to obtain the full analgesic effect, and up to three weeks to get the full anti-inflammatory effect. However, the genes you inherit affect how well NSAIDs will work for you as an individual, and around one in three of us do not notice any benefit from taking them.

Opiates (originally derived from the opium poppy) work on the nervous system to reduce the way pain signals are passed on and perceived in the brain to produce a numbing effect. Codeine is available from pharmacies to treat moderate pain and is sometimes combined with other analgesics such as aspirin, paracetamol or ibuprofen to boost their effects. Stronger opioids prescribed for long-term pain relief (e.g. dihydrocodeine, tramadol, morphine, oxycodone) only benefit around one in every four or five people and, at best, reduce pain by around 30 to 50%. For every ten people who start taking prescribed opioids for chronic pain, seven to eight will find them ineffective. If an opioid does not work within two to four weeks you are unlikely to gain more benefit with longer use.

On average, a third of people do not get significant pain relief with paracetamol, a third do not respond to codeine, and only 60% of people will respond to any NSAID.[2] This is because the genes we inherit influence how we respond and the speed at which the drug is broken down and cleared from the body (usually via the liver and kidneys).

According to an American pain survey, prescription medicines only provide effective relief in 58% of people with chronic pain.[3]

Potential side effects of conventional pain relief

Increasing numbers of people are turning to CBD supplements to treat their pain because the long-term use of paracetamol and NSAIDs is now discouraged. Concerns about potentially serious side effects, some of which have only recently become recognised, mean that doctors are now advised to prescribe the lowest effective dose of NSAIDs for the shortest period of time needed to control symptoms.

Intestinal irritation: Aspirin, ibuprofen and stronger NSAIDs only available on prescription can irritate the stomach lining and, in some cases, cause peptic ulceration. Paracetamol is now also known to do this.

Liver damage: Paracetamol (acetaminophen) is the commonest cause of acute liver failure and it is surprisingly easy to take a potentially deadly overdose of paracetamol unintentionally.

Kidney damage: NSAIDs can affect the kidneys, leading to salt and fluid retention which raises blood pressure and can lead to swelling of the ankles. People with coronary artery disease and those over the age of sixty-five years are most at risk of experiencing serious kidney problems.

Cardiovascular disease: NSAIDs cause blood pressure to increase and are linked to an increased risk of heart failure, heart attack and stroke – the greatest risk is for those taking a high dose over an extended period.

In contrast to the higher doses of aspirin used as a pain-killer, so-called mini-aspirin is prescribed in much lower doses to thin the blood and prevent unwanted clotting. However, even these low doses can irritate the stomach and cause peptic ulceration in some people.

While doctors often recommend paracetamol as a 'safer' alternative to NSAIDs such as ibuprofen, the potential side effects are similar in both with long-term use.

Opiate side effects: Most people taking opioid painkillers (such as codeine, dihydrocodeine, tramadol, oxycodone or morphine) experience at least one unwanted side effect, of which the most common are constipation and drowsiness. They are also well-known for causing addiction and, at higher doses, can suppress breathing which, in some cases, is life-threatening.

Rebound headache: If all those long-term risks aren't enough, when you stop taking painkillers such as aspirin, sinus-relief medications, paracetamol (acetaminophen), ibuprofen and codeine, you may experience a withdrawal reaction in which symptoms return with a vengeance. You may also experience a rebound headache as part of the withdrawal reaction, especially if you use painkillers more than two or three times a week on a regular basis. This is known as 'medication overuse headache' and is thought to affect up to one in fifty(2%) people worldwide.

In view of all of the above, it's not surprising that people are looking for a more natural way to help ease long-term pain.

Where CBD and the endocannabinoid system fit in

Despite rising concerns about prescription painkillers, almost one in three people experiencing pain take prescribed pain relief on a daily basis and so there has never been a greater need for an alternative, safer, pain-relieving option. The relatively recent availability of CBD supplements has added greatly to our natural painkilling armoury. The explosion of CBD products on the shelves is partly due to all the research studies and anecdotal reports that suggest it is effective in a surprisingly wide range of conditions. It appears to be especially helpful for relieving pain from a variety of causes such as migraine, arthritis, irritable bowel syndrome and fibromyalgia – health problems that are often difficult to treat with conventional medications.

As the complexities of the endocannabinoid system were unravelled, its gatekeeper role in maintaining normal immune responses and controlling pain led to a lightbulb moment. Was the newly discovered endocannabinoid system the missing link that might explain the underlying cause of the many chronic pain conditions that are resistant to conventional treatment?

This idea was first suggested in 2001 by Dr Ethan Russo, a neurologist and psychopharmacology researcher (a specialist in how drugs affect the mind).[4] Given that many brain disorders are associated with a lack of neurotransmitters (brain communication chemicals), it made sense that an equivalent lack of endocannabinoids might also lead to predictable clinical symptoms. These symptoms would be expected to involve functions in which endocannabinoids play a role, such as pain perception, the ability to relax, digestion, mood, sleep and immune reactions.

Other Conditions Caused by a Lack of Neurotransmitters

Neurotransmitters are communication chemicals released by nerve cells to pass messages to other cells. Within the brain, neurotransmitters help to control our mood and ability to think and move.

Depression is linked with a lack of neurotransmitters

such as serotonin and noradrenaline (also called norepi-nephrine) which help to regulate our mood.

Parkinson's disease is associated with a lack of the neurotransmitter dopamine, in deep parts of the brain involved in movement.

Alzheimer's disease features a lack of the neurotransmitter acetylcholine, which is needed for short-term memory and learning.

Could conditions that feature pain result from a lack of endocannabinoids that act as neurotransmitters?

This idea became known as the 'endocannabinoid deficiency' hypothesis and was first proposed in relation to migraine. It was soon extended to include other conditions that are often resistant to treatment such as fibromyalgia and irritable bowel syndrome,[5] and provided a neat explanation for why these conditions often occur together. For example, almost all (97%) people with fibromyalgia also experience headaches; over a third of people with daily headaches have symptoms that fit a diagnosis of fibromyalgia, and around a third of people with irritable bowel syndrome also have symptoms of fibromyalgia and vice versa. These close relationships strongly suggest that a similar underlying cause is involved.

While definitive proof of the endocannabinoid deficiency hypothesis is still lacking, researchers have found some supporting evidence. For example, people who suffer from migraine tend to have significantly lower than normal levels of the endocannabinoid anandamide in their cerebrospinal fluid (which bathes the brain). This is surprising given that anandamide is normally produced in greater amounts when pain is present, so lack of anandamide may be linked with migraine – although whether it is a cause or an effect is not yet known. Whichever is the case, taking CBD (which boosts anandamide levels) might be expected to help reduce the severity of symptoms.

How the endocannabinoid system regulates pain

Activation of the endocannabinoid system plays a key role in the body's response to acute and chronic pain and helps to damp down the release of neurotransmitters that control pain perception.

Endocannabinoid receptors are especially concentrated in cells that detect and respond to damage and the subsequent transmission of pain signals, including skin cells (the body's first line of protection), nerve endings that detect pain, immune cells that trigger inflammation and spinal cord cells that relay pain signals to the brain, as well as the brain cells that are involved in recognising these signals and generating feelings of pain.

When tissues anywhere in the body are injured, they produce the endocannabinoids anandamide and 2-AG. These activate our endocannabinoid receptors in the area to suppress oversensitivity and regulate the level of inflammation that results. They are able to do this because they act as 'retrograde messengers' that work backwards against the normal flow of messages to switch them off (see page 59). In other words, they return messages back to where they came from, like undelivered mail. If levels of endocannabinoids are depleted, however, the flow of messages will continue unabated. As a result, your threshold for experiencing pain is reduced and you may become overly sensitive to even mild sensations (such as a light touch) that you would not normally expect to cause pain.

If this endocannabinoid deficiency hypothesis is true, then cannabinoid supplements should help to act as a replacement so that any oversensitivity to pain returns to normal. Research is now starting to confirm this.

Clinical trials of cannabinoids for pain

Cannabis extracts have been used for centuries to relieve pain and were even referred to as a panacea, or cure-all. It's now known that cannabinoids have the best analgesic effect in conditions that are associated with inflammation and oversensitivity to pain signals – a condition known medically as hyperalgesia, which literally means 'high pain'.

Clinical trials lasting from several days to several months have found cannabis-based treatments are effective for many different types of pain associated with rheumatoid arthritis, multiple sclerosis, acute pancreatitis, HIV and chronic (long-term) pain caused by nerve damage, which is known as neuropathic pain. As a result, medical marijuana and cannabis-based pharmaceutical drugs are licensed in some countries for the treatment of pain that has not responded to other medications, which is sometimes called refractory pain.

A survey in Arizona, USA, of people using medical cannabis (CBD + THC) found that it produced significant pain relief for 77% of those with fibromyalgia, 63% with arthritis and 51% with neuropathic pain.[6]

In 2015, the *Journal of the American Medical Association* (*JAMA*) examined the results from a large number of clinical trials exploring the effectiveness of cannabinoids for a wide range of conditions. Of these, twenty-eight involved a total of 2,454 people suffering from chronic pain. The results from these studies confirmed that medical cannabis (prescribed to provide an equal blend of THC plus CBD or, in some cases, THC alone) reduced pain significantly more than placebo.[7]

A placebo is an inactive substance that is made to resemble the active treatment Researchers then compare the effects of the real treatment against the placebo. Any difference between the two helps to rule out other factors, such as improvements that naturally occur over time and the emotional benefits of being in a trial (with regular medical assessments and doctors taking your symptoms seriously).

However, a study published in the *Journal of Pain* in September 2019 suggests that patients can develop a tolerance to the use of the THC component of medical marijuana, which means it can become less effective the longer it is used so you need increasing doses. This online survey involved 989 adults who used medical marijuana (cannabis) every day, mostly for chronic pain. Those taking part were asked about how often they used it, their preferred way of using it (smoking, vaping, eating, tinctures, topical balms or other) and their preferred blends, which were divided into six different types based on the amount of CBD and THC present.[8]

The researchers classed light use as once or twice a day. Moderate use of medical marijuana was defined as three to four times per day, and heavy use as five or more times per day.

Interestingly, those who were light users and those who favoured products high in CBD tended to have a greater improvement in symptoms than those who preferred higher levels of THC. Overall, increased frequency of medical marijuana use and higher intakes of THC were associated with worse pain (which could mean that the benefits of THC were wearing off) and worse side effects, such as fatigue and sleep disturbances. The researchers suggested that the more marijuana is used by people with chronic pain, the more tolerant they become to its effects. If they then take higher doses to obtain the same effects, they are more likely to experience side effects. Finding the right balance is key.[9]

This is further supported by a small trial involving fifteen healthy (and brave) volunteers who agreed to have a chilli extract (capsaicin) injected under their skin to trigger burning pain. They then smoked marijuana from cigarettes providing different amounts of THC and the results were compared with smoking a placebo cigarette containing no THC. Smoking a low-dose cigarette (providing 2% THC) offered no relief against the pain, smoking a medium-dose cigarette (containing 4% THC) did provide significant pain relief, but smoking a high-dose cigarette (with 8% THC) actually *increased* pain perception. This suggests that THC produces a Goldilocks effect – you need just the right amount; too little doesn't work and too much can have the opposite effect you are looking for.

CBD for pain

Despite surveys showing that pain is the most common reason why people choose to take CBD extracts, there have been few clinical trials assessing the effects of CBD in people with long-term pain. This is mostly due to the historically restrictive legal status of cannabis which created a lot of paperwork for researchers wanting to carry out clinical trials.

Now that CBD is more widely used, it is emerging as an analgesic in its own right. However, good quality clinical trials can cost hundreds of thousands of pounds – more than small manufacturers of CBD products are able to invest, so almost all trials are carried out by pharmaceutical companies who have created virtually pure (isolate, or narrow spectrum) CBD-based drugs rather than CBD oils that include other cannabinoids naturally found in hemp plants (broad spectrum, or full spectrum, see page 94). This allows them to patent their particular extract to help recoup the cost of their investment in research.

Another factor that discourages small manufacturers from carrying out research is that if they want their CBD product to be associated with claims relating to pain relief, they would have to position it as a medicine rather than a food supplement. The product would then have to undergo all the additional legal requirements associated with pharmaceutical medicines and, assuming it passed, it would then only be available on prescription rather than freely available as a supplement.

Even so, a small study from Uruguay (the first country in the world to legalise recreational marijuana alongside medical marijuana) was published in 2018.[10] This study involved seven people with chronic pain following a kidney transplant who wanted to use CBD for pain relief. Their doctors prescribed CBD at an initial dose of 100mg per day, which was progressively increased, as needed, up to 300mg per day (this dose should only be used under medical supervision). Two out of the seven patients reported total pain relief and another four had a good response – only one patient did not notice any reduction in pain with CBD.

Because of the lack of evidence, NHS doctors in England are currently advised not to prescribe CBD to manage chronic pain (unless as part of a clinical trial) by NICE (the National Institute for Health and Care Excellence, whose guidelines advise doctors on what drugs to prescribe for different conditions based on cost and effectiveness). Elsewhere, doctors are listening to patients who find CBD helpful and some now recommend it for pain relief. Writing in the journal *Pain and Therapy* in 2019, for example, two US pain specialists indicated that they now use CBD oil to treat some patients with chronic pain as part of their overall strategy and have found it provides great benefit.[11] However, they then go on to underline the importance of taking good quality, trustworthy CBD products, and the need for regulations to ensure accurate labelling of CBD oil products.

See chapter five for guidance on how to select a safe CBD product.

IMPORTANT Many people don't think to tell their doctor that they are taking herbal medicines or other natural supplements. If you have a medical condition, always talk to your doctor before taking CBD. It is important to check if CBD interacts with any medicines you are taking, whether prescribed or bought from a pharmacy, including paracetamol (acetaminophen), ibuprofen or codeine.

CBD interacts with the enzymes in the liver that break down many drugs, including painkillers. This can increase blood levels of your medicine (so you are more likely to experience side effects) or, in some cases, lower levels of your medicine (so it becomes less effective).

How CBD relieves pain

The exact way in which CBD suppresses pain remains uncertain, although there are lots of plausible theories based on laboratory studies.

Back in 1988, it was suggested that there was a specific cannabinoid pain receptor in the brain. This is now known not to be the case. Instead, researchers have found at least sixty-five different ways in which CBD can interact with our cells, including at least ten different types of receptor. These include the two specific cannabinoid receptors (CB1 and CB2, see chapter three) plus opioid receptors (involved in pain relief) and serotonin receptors (which help to regulate mood). CBD also affects the way certain substances move across cell membranes (e.g. neurotransmitters, which pass pain messages in the brain), the flow of electrolytes in and out of cells (e.g. calcium, magnesium and sodium, which can improve how cells work and ensure their survival) and the action of over thirty specific enzymes – proteins that are vital for certain chemical reactions to occur.[12]

Its wide range of actions results from the way CBD interacts with immune cells, sensory nerves, the spinal cord and the brain. In fact, CBD can produce painkilling benefits through a combination of different effects, such as prolonging the effects of anandamide (one of our natural endocannabinoids), inhibiting the release of inflammatory molecules (e.g. prostaglandins), stimulating the release of natural painkillers (e.g. endorphins), relaxing muscle spasms, damping down the transmission of pain signals, raising pain thresholds and enhancing the effects of natural brain neurotransmitters (such as serotonin and dopamine). These actions all have positive effects on how pain signals are interpreted. What's more, as CBD works in so many different ways, it is likely to be effective in most people – even if the genes you inherit weaken one of its actions, it can still work in other ways to provide some benefits.

In addition, CBD is an antioxidant that is more powerful than vitamin C or vitamin E in suppressing inflammation and protecting nerve fibres from damage.

So, CBD not only reduces the number and level of pain signals triggered, it alters the way you respond to them and helps you feel and cope much better. The ability of CBD to reduce anxiety and stress, lift mood and improve sleep has a positive effect on our perception of pain. And it does all of this without the 'high' associated with medical marijuana or the potentially serious side effects of pharmaceutical painkilling drugs.

CB2 receptors within the central nervous system are normally scarce but their number increases as your level of pain intensifies, so CBD becomes more effective.

Using CBD for pain

If you have pain, have seen your doctor and know what is causing it, you may decide to try a CBD oil instead of standard painkillers. If you don't know the cause of your pain, however, do see your doctor first in case you need any tests or other medical treatments.

Chapter five explains the different types of CBD supplements available, how to select a quality product and use it safely (for example by checking that CBD does not affect and will not interact with any other medicines you are taking). Many people find they get the best pain relief from a full-spectrum CBD oil that contains small amounts of all the other cannabinoids normally present within hemp plants, as these act together to produce more wide-ranging effects. Others may respond best to a broad-spectrum CBD supplement that has had the THC removed. Everyone is different, however, and you may find that a narrow-spectrum supplement that provides mostly pure CBD (having had most or all of the other cannabinoids removed) suits you best. You may need to try several different supplements and increasing doses to find what works best for you.

As pain is subjective, it's difficult for others to understand the level of discomfort you are experiencing. It is also difficult to remember what pain feels like yourself, once it has reduced in severity or gone away completely. To help assess how well your pain is responding to CBD, it's a good idea to keep a pain diary for at least the first few weeks that you are taking CBD, to record the level of pain you are experiencing each day.

Pain is usually rated on a scale of 0 to 10, where 0 means no pain and 10 means the worst pain imaginable. You may find it easiest to do this using a scale like the one overleaf. With a ruler, draw a series of lines about 10 centimetres long. Looking back through your marked lines will help you to see at a glance whether your pain is reducing as a result of using CBD oil supplements.

As explained in chapter five, the speed at which CBD works will depend on the type of supplement you use and the dose you take. Oral sprays and CBD oil drops held in the mouth for a couple of minutes will speed its absorption into your bloodstream. Capsules taken by mouth will work more slowly. You should notice some pain relief from a single dose, usually within twenty minutes to an hour, with the maximum effect usually occurring within two to three hours. Regular use, taking CBD two or three times a day (depending on the manufacturer's instructions), should help to keep pain at bay.

If treating a temporary form of pain, such as a headache or sprain, you can stop using CBD as soon as your symptoms get better. If you have long-term (chronic) pain (for example, due to osteoarthritis) or pain that comes and goes (e.g. due to irritable bowel syndrome) you may need to take CBD long term, too. If your pain is linked with an endocannabinoid deficiency (see earlier in this chapter), then taking CBD may help to restore balance and allow your body to start making the correct amounts of endocannabinoids again. To find out if this is the case, once your pain improves stop taking CBD to see if the pain recurs. If your pain persists, speak to your doctor to see what they recommend.

Each day, simply mark an X along the length of the scale to represent the level of pain you experienced within the previous twenty-four hours. For example:

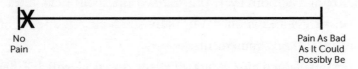

This line represents a good day with hardly any pain.

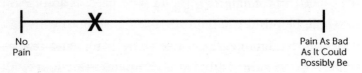

This line shows a day on which someone experienced mild to moderate pain (about 3 on a 0 to 10 scale).

Headache pain

Headaches are among the most common reasons for taking CBD supplements.

Although you may think that all headaches are the same,

there are over a hundred different types with a variety of different causes and symptoms. Of these, tension headaches are the most common (accounting for 40% of headaches), followed by migraine (10%), which affects at least 700 million people worldwide. CBD can help both these common types of headache, and a more rare and severe form known as cluster headaches. So far, these are the only three types of headache researchers have studied for the effects of CBD.

A tension headache is usually mild to moderate in intensity and typically feels like a steady, continuous pressure, or a tight, constricting band over the top and back of your head, or over both eyes. This type of headache is associated with stress and is due to tension in your neck and scalp muscles (partly caused by the way you hold yourself when stressed), which affects blood flow within the skull.

A migraine is a severe pain that is usually (but not always) worse on one side of the head, producing a severe, throbbing, pulsating or hammering headache along with nausea, vomiting, sensitivity to light and sound. Around one in ten people with migraine experience warning signs (known as an aura) in the form of visual symptoms such as shimmering or flashing lights, strange zigzag shapes or blind spots before the pain begins in earnest. The exact cause of migraine is not yet fully understood, but is believed to involve inflammation that causes overstimulation of the trigeminal nerve (the largest of the twelve cranial nerves in the head) and changes in blood flow within parts of the brain. Increasing evidence suggests this is all linked with lower than normal levels of the natural endocannabinoid anandamide, which lowers the threshold at which inflammation leads to pain.[13]

A cluster headache is one of the most severe types of pain you can experience – so bad it is also known as a 'suicide headache'. One eye becomes congested and watery, the nostril on the same side is usually blocked, and you may experience facial sweating, flushing and swelling of the eyelid. The pain lasts for up to three hours and comes on regularly – usually at the same time of day and often in the early morning, waking you from sleep – for one to three weeks before disappearing. Although sufferers are perfectly well between attacks, the pain is so severe that many live in fear of the next one occurring. While the cause of cluster headaches is unknown, it may involve over-activation of a part of the brain due to lower than normal levels of natural endocannabinoids. If this is the case, then taking CBD may be expected to help.

Headaches

The following are some of the more common medically recognised triggers for headaches: sexual activity, coughing, excess sleep (more than eight hours) when you are not accustomed to it, such as at the weekend, caffeine withdrawal, rebound effect of paracetamol or ibuprofen (see page 129), alcohol, food sensitivities (e.g. monosodium glutamate, or MSG), premenstrual hormone swings, eating ice cream or other very cold foods and inhaling strong perfumes.

CBD is believed to reduce the symptoms and frequency of headaches in several different ways. As well as activating cannabinoid receptors, it also has positive effects on serotonin, opiate and other receptors known to influence the transmission and perception of pain signals. Its antioxidant effects within the brain may also damp down the over-production of inflammatory chemicals linked with migraine headaches, as well as suppressing the overactivity of a type of brain cell known as microglia. Microglia are scavenging cells that wander around the brain clearing up unwanted debris. They secrete up to twenty times more of the painkilling endo-cannabinoid anandamide than other brain cells, and carry both CB1 and CB2 receptors. Microglia that are overactive can cause inflammation and are believed to play a role in a variety of neurological diseases, including migraines that are accompanied by a warning aura.

A large and growing body of research suggests that a lack of endocannabinoids may be implicated in many different types of headache, and that treatment with plant cannabinoids can help to prevent and treat them. As we have seen, the conventional treatment for headaches – paracetamol, aspirin and non-steroidal anti-inflammatory drugs (NSAIDs) such as ibuprofen – do not work for around one in three people. Drugs known as triptans are also used at onset to help prevent migraine and cluster headaches taking hold, but one in four people who experience migraines do not respond to triptans and, of those who do, only a third remain pain-free after two hours, and only one in five remain pain-free for twenty-four hours.[14] This is why many people are turning to alternative treatments such a medical marijuana and CBD.

What the research shows

The past classification of cannabis products as Schedule 1 drugs has stifled research into the medical benefits of phytocannabinoids. As a result, no gold-standard, placebo-controlled clinical trials have been carried out using either medical marijuana or CBD alone to treat headaches. There are some patient surveys and small studies that show promising results, however.

Two clinics in Colorado that prescribed medical marijuana for 121 people with migraine found it more than halved the number of migraines (from 10.4 attacks per month down to 4.6). To achieve this, most patients used more than one form of marijuana, however, and had to use it daily.[15]

Another interesting study, which was presented at the Third Congress of the European Academy of Neurology in Amsterdam in June 2017, suggests that cannabinoids are just as effective in preventing migraines as other treatments. Forty-eight people with chronic migraine or cluster headaches were given 10mg of an oral medical marijuana preparation that contained twice as much THC (19%) as CBD (9%). This dose did not prevent migraines so was slowly increased up to a daily dose of 100mg, which did help to reduce the number of migraines. When an attack occurred, taking an extra dose of 200mg of the medical marijuana reduced the intensity of pain by more than half.[16] (NB Only take these high doses with the permission of your doctor.)

In a later study, the effects of taking 200mg per day of this THC–CBD blend for three months were compared with a daily dose of 25mg amitriptyline (an antidepressant sometimes used to reduce migraine pain). Another group of people with cluster headaches also took part in the study and received either 200mg of the THC–CBD combination per day, or a conventional treatment (the calcium channel blocker drug, verapamil). In all cases, anyone who developed a migraine was also asked to take an additional dose of the 200mg TCH–CBD combination.

At the end of the study, the results showed that the cannabinoid combination was slightly better than amitriptyline for treating migraines, reducing the number of attacks by 40.1% and their severity by 43.5%. In those with cluster headaches, however, the medical marijuana only seemed to work in people with cluster headache who had previously experienced migraine in childhood. The overall conclusion was that cannabinoids are an effective alternative treatment for preventing migraines, although, as always, more studies are needed to confirm this.

In the case of CBD, surveys carried out by manufacturers suggest that many people find CBD supplements helpful for reducing headaches but there is not yet enough clinical trial evidence to confirm this one way or the other. The only way to know if CBD will help you, as an individual, is to try it. If you are receiving medical treatment for your headaches, do talk to your doctor first, and check whether there are any known interactions with the medicines you are taking.

Try massaging a little CBD salve into your temples to relieve a tension headache.

It is particularly important to seek medical advice if you are experiencing:

- A severe, sudden-onset headache
- A headache that keeps getting worse and won't go away, or which changes dramatically
- Three or more headaches a week
- Other symptoms such as a fever, stiff neck, rash, vomiting, confusion, drowsiness or unexpected symptoms affecting the eyes, ears, nose or throat
- Headache plus dizziness, slurred speech, weakness, or changes in sensation (numbness and/or tingling)
- A headache following a head injury
- A headache triggered by exertion, coughing or bending
- Headaches during pregnancy (to rule out pre-eclampsia in which blood pressure is high)

These symptoms are red flags for potentially serious types of headache that require further investigation and treatment.

Irritable bowel syndrome pain

There is now good evidence that irritable bowel syndrome (IBS) is associated with a deficiency in the endocannabinoid system.[17] If this is the case, then a CBD supplement may help to reduce the symptoms of IBS, such as abdominal pain or discomfort, bloating and a change in bowel habit (diarrhoea, constipation or both). In this case, I suggest using CBD in the form of capsules, an oral spray or drops, however, as the sweeteners added to some gummies (e.g. agave syrup, high-fructose corn syrup, molasses, isomalt, sorbitol, maltitol, xylitol) may worsen IBS symptoms in some people. Gummies sweetened with stevia, sugar or sucralose are less likely to cause problems.

IBS is the most common condition affecting the gut and it accounts for up to half of visits to GPs for gastrointestinal complaints. According to the International Foundation for Gastrointestinal Disorders, IBS affects between one in ten and one in six of us (10 to 15% of the global population).

IBS has proven notoriously difficult to treat and is now recognised as not just a problem of bowel function but the result of faulty communication between the gut and brain. Normally, the brain filters out all the sensations involved with digestion, such as the bowel contractions that propel solid wastes downwards, so these do not reach the level of conscious thought. When you have IBS, however, these sensations are not filtered out as well as normal, and the signals produced by oversensitive stretch receptors in the gut lining get through to the brain where they are perceived as pain.

An interesting study looked at the human genes that provide the blueprint for making the different parts of our endocannabinoid system. When comparing these genes in people with IBS with those in healthy volunteers, they found that inheriting some variations of these genes increased the risk of developing IBS, diarrhoea and increased pain sensitivity in parts of the large bowel.[18] This suggests that the endocannabinoid system is closely linked with irritable bowel syndrome, and it is now thought that an oversensitivity to gut sensations may be due to an endocannabinoid deficiency.

This is not the whole story, however, and the types of bacteria living in our large bowel are also believed to be important.

Of the more than 1,000 species of bacteria that commonly live on and in the human body, we each harbour a unique mix of around 150 different types within our gut. While some of these species are found in most people, we each have our own specific blend of gut bacteria that is as individual as our fingerprints. Our unique blend of bacteria is now thought to affect our susceptibility to conditions such as irritable bowel syndrome. The total number of these bacteria is greater than our personal total of human cells, and they contain a wider variety of genes than the 23,000 human ones we each possess, making each of us, arguably, more bacterial than human!

These bacteria make thousands of bacterial proteins, whose hormonal, enzyme and inflammatory actions can affect our normal gut function. In fact, approximately 10% of the activity of human genes within the intestinal wall is believed to be regulated by the microbes present. This includes interactions with our endocannabinoid system, which might affect whether or not we experience symptoms of IBS.

Bacterial Imbalances

An imbalance in the types of bacteria within the gut (known as dysbiosis) can trigger IBS symptoms. This can follow a bout of food poisoning, taking antibiotics, long-term stress or surgery. These imbalances include the loss of beneficial 'probiotic' bacteria (which produce lactic acid and natural antibiotics to suppress the less desirable, gas-forming bacteria). This results in the overgrowth of

less beneficial bacteria and increased fermentation, leading to abdominal discomfort, bloating and changes in
bowel habit such as diarrhoea or constipation.

Bacteria are now believed to have indirect effects on our
brain through their interactions with endocannabinoid
receptors and serotonin within the gut wall. Serotonin is
best known as a brain transmitter that regulates mood, but
95% of our serotonin is actually made within the lining
of our digestive tract. Within the gut, serotonin appears
to regulate bowel movements and the way in, which the
brain usually ignores the sensations caused by normal gut
contractions.

Our gut, immune system and brain are in constant communication through the complex network of nerves found
within our intestines. This network (the enteric nervous
system) is sometimes referred to as our 'second brain', as it
works independently of the autonomic nervous system that
regulates our other automatic body functions such as our
heart rate and breathing.

The nerves and immune cells within the gut wall are
richly endowed with endocannabinoid receptors that
help to regulate intestinal movements and the secretion
of intestinal juices, as well as controlling inflammation.
Researchers now believe that gut bacteria can activate these
endocannabinoid receptors to inhibit bowel contractions,
for example, leading to constipation.

All these new understandings are helping to explain the
underlying cause of irritable bowel syndrome and why its

symptoms are often worse during times of physical and emotional stress.

A Traditional Cholera Cure

In 1840, a preparation of Indian hemp (*Cannabis indica*) was declared a promising treatment for the intense watery diarrhoea associated with cholera.

What the research shows

Researchers have suggested that taking plant cannabinoids such as CBD might reduce the symptoms of irritable bowel syndrome and other intestinal problems by boosting levels of anandamide (to overcome an endocannabinoid deficiency).[19] CBD may also work in other ways as it is known to interact with a non-cannabinoid receptor called TRPV1, which is involved in feeling pain. Biopsies show that people with IBS have 3.5 times more of these receptors in their intestinal nerves as people without IBS.[20]

Several studies have looked at how THC affects our bowel function. In healthy volunteers, a single dose of a synthetic form of THC relaxed the colon and reduced contractions after eating. Unexpectedly, however, THC was found to increase pain perception when the colon was distended (by inserting a balloon).[21] This suggests that THC may increase the sensitivity of stretch receptors, which could make IBS symptoms worse in some cases. Other studies have found that THC did not reduce IBS pain or diarrhoea.[22] [23] Together, these findings seem to rule out using high-THC forms of medical marijuana to ease IBS symptoms, but what about CBD alone?

Frustratingly, no one has yet funded and published any clinical trials into the effects of cannabidiol when used to treat irritable bowel syndrome. All we really have to go on are anecdotal reports from IBS forums and user surveys suggesting that CBD does improve IBS symptoms by relaxing bowel spasms and reducing cramps, pain and diarrhoea. The evidence from laboratory studies also suggests it should work, but we don't yet have the clinical trials to prove that CBD is an effective treatment for IBS.

The only way to know if CBD can help your symptoms, based on your individual genes and unique bowel bacterial balance, is to try it and see how you respond.

IMPORTANT Don't diagnose irritable bowel syndrome yourself and always seek medical advice if you experience recurrent abdominal pain, bloating or a change in bowel habit.

Fibromyalgia pain

Fibromyalgia is another long-term pain disorder that is thought to result from an endocannabinoid deficiency. If this is the case, CBD may help to ease the symptoms for as long as it is taken. Whether or not CBD will act like a reset button to restore more normal activity within the endocannabinoid system remains to be seen.

Fibromyalgia is an unpleasant condition that causes widespread pain. One of its hallmarks is the presence of specific tender points on the body that hurt when pressure is applied. Typically, something that others might perceive as touch is instead experienced as pain. FMRI (functional magnetic resonance imaging) studies have shown that, in fibromyalgia, mild pressure 'lights up' parts of the brain that normally only respond to pain. As a result, fibromyalgia is now thought of as a centralised pain state, meaning that it involves the central nervous system which does not process pain signals properly.

Fibromyalgia affects an estimated 5.4% of the UK population. Two out of three people diagnosed with fibromyalgia are female and women usually have more tender points than men, although the reason is unknown.

Studies involving twins suggest that around half the risk of developing fibromyalgia and related pain conditions (such as irritable bowel syndrome and migraine) is genetic, while half is related to environmental triggers such as stress, exposure to certain infections (e.g. Lyme disease) or to severe trauma (e.g. motor accidents, surgery).[24]

A musical metaphor has been used to liken the degree of pain felt in centralised pain conditions such as fibromyalgia to the loudness of an electric guitar. Before the signals produced by the guitar strings (equivalent to sensory nerves) can be heard, the information must first pass through an amplifier – in this case, the brain. For most of us, pain is felt when the strings (nerves) are plucked harder and faster, but for those with a centralised pain state, the intensity is instead due to turning up the amplifier. This amplification makes all the 'strings' louder so that pain becomes impossible to ignore.[25]

The pain associated with fibromyalgia often comes and goes in different parts of the body and can be accompanied by feelings of numbness, tingling or burning. Other possible symptoms include oversensitivity to bright lights, loud noises or smells, plus fatigue, memory problems, difficulty thinking straight, headaches, sleep disturbances and low mood.

As well as increased sensitivity to pain, people with fibromyalgia also experience poor quality sleep with less time spent in the refreshing REM (rapid eye movement, or dreaming) phase of sleep. They also often wake more after falling asleep, and spend more time in the light stages of sleep and less time in deep sleep than normal.

These symptoms and findings are all consistent with what you would expect if there were an underlying endocannabinoid deficiency.

CBD has the potential to improve many, if not all, of the symptoms of fibromyalgia by reducing pain, relieving anxiety, lifting mood and increasing time spent in refreshing REM sleep.

A number of medical treatments are used to help relieve fibromyalgia, including stress reduction programmes, cognitive behavioural therapy (CBT), structured exercise regimes, conventional painkillers and drugs that help to normalise pain perception (some of which are also used as antidepressants or anticonvulsants).

Painkillers such as non-steroidal anti-inflammatory drugs (NSAIDs such as ibuprofen) and paracetamol are not particularly effective in treating chronic pain conditions and are also limited by their side effects when used over a long time (see pages 127–8). Opiate painkillers are best avoided as, paradoxically, they appear to worsen sensitivity to pain in people with fibromyalgia (an effect known as opioid-induced hyperalgesia).[26]

What the research shows

Given that many people now think that fibromyalgia may be linked to an endocannabinoid deficiency, a few clinical trials are starting to assess the effects of cannabinoid treatment using medical marijuana products containing different combinations of THC and CBD.

One study that looked at the effects of medical marijuana in people with fibromyalgia found the proportion of patients who reported strong relief from their symptoms ranged from 81% in the case of sleep problems, down to 14% when it came to headaches. However, almost all users (twenty-seven out of twenty-eight) reported unwanted side effects such as dry mouth, sedation, dizziness, a drug 'high', eye irritation or rapid pulse.[27]

Another recent study, published in April 2019, explored the analgesic effects of different strengths of inhaled (vaped) medical marijuana in twenty people with fibromyalgia.[28] The four blends used contained either high THC (22.4mg) with virtually no CBD (less than 1mg); high CBD (17.8mg) and high THC (13.4mg); high CBD (18.4mg) with virtually no THC (less than 1mg); or no THC and no CBD (to act as a placebo).

After a single inhalation, significantly more people using the product that was high in both CBD and THC experienced at least a 30% decrease in pressure pain compared to placebo. On its own, pure CBD did not seem to be any more effective than the placebo, but this may have been because only a single dose of each of the inhaled cannabinoids was tested; other studies have found that people battling chronic pain often only experience a small analgesic response after a single inhalation. Regular use is needed to obtain good relief from chronic pain that has been present for some time. Further studies are therefore needed to determine the effects of longer treatment with CBD for pain relief.

Although it is early days in terms of research, anecdotal reports and surveys suggest that CBD oil alone does help to relieve the symptoms of fibromyalgia such as pain and sleep disturbances. The only way to know if it will suit you as an individual is to try it. Talk to your doctor first and read the chapter on using CBD safely.

Diverticular disease pain

Diverticular disease may also be linked to an endocannabinoid deficiency within the large bowel. If this is the case, then CBD supplements would be expected to improve the pain and other symptoms experienced by sufferers.

Diverticular disease develops when small 'blow outs' from

the lining of the colon push through the outer muscle of the bowel wall to form pouches that protrude from the bowel's surface. Several of these sac-like protrusions form and usually measure from 5mm to 10mm across.

Diverticular disease becomes increasingly common over the age of forty and affects as many as one in two people over the age of sixty.

While most people are unaware they are affected, these pouches can cause symptoms such as a change in bowel habit (diarrhoea, constipation), nausea, flatulence, bloating and pain. Discomfort is usually worse in the lower, left-hand side of the abdomen where the affected part of the large bowel is located. The pouches can also become infected and inflamed when filled with trapped bowel contents (known as diverticulitis).

Diverticulosis is the presence of bowel protrusions (diverticula) that do not cause symptoms and are relatively harmless.

Diverticular disease is diagnosed when the protrusions cause intermittent lower abdominal pain but no inflammation.

Diverticulitis occurs when the protrusions become infected and inflamed, causing severe lower abdominal pain, fever and, sometimes, rectal bleeding.

The traditional view is that diverticulosis is the result of increased pressure in the bowel; for example, as a result of straining when constipated. This pushes the bowel lining through natural openings in the overlying muscular bowel wall along which blood vessels pass. Being unfit, overweight and lacking fibre in your diet increases the risk of developing the disease.

The conventional medical treatment of diverticular disease usually involves following a high-fibre diet, drinking plenty of fluids and taking laxatives to reduce the constipation that often occurs when the protrusions interfere with normal bowel contraction. If diverticulitis develops, antibiotics are prescribed to help clear the infection. In severe cases, it might be necessary to go to hospital, and complications such as abscess, bowel obstruction or perforation may mean surgery.

The use of conventional painkillers to treat diverticular disease is discouraged as aspirin, opiates such as codeine (which also worsen constipation) and NSAID painkillers have been found to increase the risk of bowel perforation.[29]

New findings, however, suggest that the formation of pouches in the bowel may actually result from faulty nerve control that affects how the bowel contracts. These contractions are partly regulated by the endocannabinoid system and researchers have now suggested that diverticulosis may be caused by reduced sensitivity of endocannabinoid receptors within the bowel wall. If this is the case, then CBD may help to stop the symptoms becoming worse.

What the research shows

It has been known for centuries that cannabis can have a beneficial effect on the gut. So far, no clinical trials have assessed the effects of CBD in alleviating the symptoms of diverticular disease; however, the results from preclinical (laboratory) studies suggest that taking CBD supplements may help.

Researchers have tested colon muscle cells obtained from people undergoing bowel surgery, comparing those collected from people with diverticular disease; to those obtained from people with bowel cancer. Our natural endocannabinoids, such as anandamide, are known to suppress bowel contractions and, in people with diverticular disease, the level of anandamide was more than twice as high as in cells from people with bowel cancer.[30] The levels of a receptor (TRPV1) with which anandamide can interact were also higher and also appeared to act abnormally in people with diverticular disease. Rather than relaxing when a known nerve blocker (tetrodotoxin derived from pufferfish) was added, the cells instead contracted more strongly. This suggests that the nerve control of colon contraction is profoundly altered in people with diverticular disease and that the endocannabinoid system is involved.

As cannabidiol interacts with CB2 receptors in the immune and nervous systems, it would be expected to suppress both the pain and inflammation associated with diverticular disease and diverticulitis. Unfortunately, no studies have yet been carried out to confirm this. As always, if you decide to try a CBD supplement to help relieve pain from diverticular disease, check with your doctor first.

Probiotic supplements containing bowel-friendly bacteria have been shown to help relieve abdominal pain and other symptoms in those with diverticular disease who also follow a high-fibre diet.[31] These may partly work by stimulating more normal function of endocannabinoid receptors in the bowel.

Inflammatory bowel disease pain

Inflammatory bowel diseases are believed to occur when immune cells mistake a normal part of the body as 'foreign' and mount an attack against it. This causes a range of severe and unpleasant symptoms including fever, abdominal pain, nausea and vomiting, diarrhoea (which may contain pus and mucus) and rectal bleeding. Not surprisingly, this can lead to poor appetite with weight loss and signs of malnutrition. Symptoms can flare up from time to time, which is known as a relapse, and these relapses may alternate with periods of being relatively symptom free (known as remissions).

Crohn's disease is a chronic (long-term) inflammatory disease in which the full thickness of the intestinal wall becomes inflamed. Only discrete parts of the gut are affected, however – anywhere from the mouth (part of the intestinal tract) to the anal canal, with apparently normal areas of bowel in between. In contrast, ulcerative colitis is an inflammatory disease of the gastrointestinal tract that mainly affects the lining (rather than the full thickness) of the rectum and a variable length of the colon. Occasionally, it's not clear which type of inflammatory bowel disease is present as features from both conditions are present. In these cases 'indeterminate colitis' is usually diagnosed.

In the UK, Crohn's disease affects at least 115,000 people. Ulcerative colitis is more common, and is thought to affect around 146,000 people.

These serious inflammatory bowel diseases may result from abnormal immune responses to the presence of certain food proteins, or the presence of certain intestinal viruses, yeasts, fungi or bacteria – although the exact causes or triggers remain unknown.

Whatever it is that sets them off, immune cells respond by releasing chemical alarm signals (cytokines) that cause tiny blood vessels in the intestinal wall to dilate, bringing in more white blood cells which secrete more inflammatory signals to escalate the attack. The resulting cascade of reactions irritates nerve endings, causing pain and inflammation that damages the bowel wall.

The current recommended medical treatment of inflammatory bowel disease involves specialist anti-inflammatory drugs such as aminosalicylates, corticosteroids and other immunosuppressive drugs in order to dampen down the abnormal immune responses described above. However, between 30 and 40% of patients do not respond to these drugs and there is an urgent need for new medicines to treat inflammatory bowel diseases.[32] Even when these drugs are effective, they are often accompanied by numerous unpleasant side effects such as nausea, diarrhoea, headaches and skin rashes so that 30 to 45% of people with inflammatory bowel disease do not take them as often as prescribed.

What the research shows

Medical marijuana and CBD alone are now undergoing clinical trials as promising new treatments for inflammatory bowel disease. If they are found to be effective, their possible side effects may be less troublesome than those associated with current treatments.

Cannabinoids could have numerous beneficial effects against inflammatory bowel disease as they help to regulate the natural interactions between immune cells and the nervous system and suppress the overactivity that can lead to unwanted inflammation, excessive bowel contractions and pain. For example, activation of CB1 cannabinoid receptors within the gut (by our own endocannabinoids) can decrease intestinal secretions and excessive intestinal contractions as well as increasing bowel leakiness in response to inflammation. On the other hand, activating CB2 receptors helps to damp down overactive immune responses and reduce intestinal leakiness caused by inflammation so that healing can occur. Producing the wrong amounts of our natural endocannabinoids may therefore lead to worsening bowel symptoms.

Laboratory studies show that adding CBD or THC to intestinal cell cultures helps to overcome leakiness caused by inflammation, allowing cells to recover their normal barrier function.[33]

Researchers have suggested that CBD is a particularly promising treatment for inflammatory bowel diseases. It helps to reduce the abnormal immune reactions that cause immune cells (neutrophils and macrophages) to move into areas of inflammation where they mount an attack that can make symptoms worse.

Good quality clinical trials are needed to confirm this, although early indications from small trials involving medical marijuana and CBD alone are positive, as described in the following pages.

Medical marijuana and inflammatory bowel disease

Over a century ago, cannabis was used to treat pain, diarrhoea and inflammation until marijuana became outlawed. In countries where medical marijuana is legal, it remains a popular self-help treatment for inflammatory bowel disease. In Canada, for example, which allowed the use of medical marijuana in 2001, around half of patients attending a specialist outpatient inflammatory bowel disease clinic had used medical cannabis at some time, and 12% with ulcerative colitis and 16% with Crohn's disease were current users. Between a third and a half said it relieved abdominal pain, diarrhoea and improved their appetite. Marijuana appeared to be especially popular to help treat pain after abdominal surgery and to help those with chronic abdominal pain get more enjoyment from life.[34]

In a small clinical trial, thirteen people with long-standing inflammatory bowel disease were prescribed inhaled medical marijuana. After three months' treatment, patients reported significant improvements in their general health and said they were better able to take part in social events and worked more effectively, due to reduced physical pain and depression. They also gained weight.

Another study assessed the effects of medical marijuana on symptoms and the need for medication in thirty people with Crohn's disease. On average, the severity of their symptoms halved and their need for other medication and even surgery was significantly reduced.[35]

But what about CBD used alone?

CBD and ulcerative colitis

One trial tested the anti-inflammatory effects of CBD in sixty people with ulcerative colitis who were on a stable dose of standard medication. Around half were given a 50mg CBD extract while the remainder took only a placebo to compare the effects. Over the course of two weeks, doses were slowly increased to the maximum amount each person could tolerate (without side effects) with the aim of reaching a dose of 250mg twice a day for ten weeks. (NB These high doses should *only* be used under medical supervision.)

Those taking CBD needed, on average, one third fewer CBD capsules than those on placebo, suggesting they were effective, and the severity of symptoms and overall quality of life improved significantly more with CBD than with placebo.

The researchers concluded that the CBD-rich extracts may be beneficial for treating the symptoms of ulcerative colitis and that larger trials are warranted.[36]

CBD and Crohn's disease

A small trial published in 2017 suggests that CBD is not effective in treating Crohn's disease.[37]

This particular trial used a pure CBD product (99.5%) dissolved in olive oil, so there were no other cannabinoids present to boost its action (see entourage effect, page 23). Nineteen people with active Crohn's disease that had not responded to standard medical treatment were given either CBD (at a low dose of just 10mg) twice a day, or a placebo, for eight weeks. In those taking cannabidiol, the severity of symptoms reduced from a score of 337 down to 220; however, this was not statistically significant compared with placebo. Having said that, those who were randomly assigned to take CBD had much worse symptoms to start with (a score of 337 compared with 308) so their improvement was impressive. The dose of CBD used was also unusually small (just 10mg taken twice a day), there was no entourage effect and the duration of the study was quite short (eight weeks). As the researchers themselves pointed out, larger studies are needed, using higher doses of CBD (from plant extracts rather than just isolated CBD) and for a longer period of time, before its use is dismissed.

If you have inflammatory bowel disease, always talk to your doctor before starting to take a CBD supplement, and check for interactions with any drugs you are taking.

Some varieties of probiotic bacteria prevent a flare-up (relapse) of inflammatory bowel diseases and help symptoms fade away. These probiotic bacteria may partly work by stimulating the endocannabinoid system within the bowel wall to improve leakiness and suppress unwanted immune reactions.

Endometriosis pain

Many women find CBD helpful for reducing period pains and the more severe menstrual cramps that are associated with endometriosis.

Endometriosis is the only known condition in which apparently normal, non-cancerous cells spread from one part of the body (the womb lining or endometrium) to another, most commonly within the pelvic or abdominal cavities, where they take root and continue to grow. These misplaced cells are still sensitive to the monthly hormone cycle, which means they can swell and bleed into surrounding tissues once a month, just as they would in the lining of the womb. This causes pain, inflammation and scarring, which produces patches (or lesions) outside of the uterus. Symptoms of endometriosis include heavy, painful periods, pain during sex and deep pelvic pain (which can occur throughout the menstrual cycle). One in three women will also experience difficulty conceiving.

Overall, around one in ten women of reproductive age have endometriosis, rising to one in three of all women experiencing fertility problems and one in two women with severe period pains and chronic pelvic pain (whose endometriosis often goes undiagnosed). There is no obvious link between the severity of symptoms and the extent of lesions seen during laparoscopy (key-hole surgery), however. In some women, minimal signs of disease can cause maximum pain and distress. Other women with extensive, widespread disease may have no symptoms and be unaware they are affected.

The current recommended treatment for endometriosis includes non-steroidal anti-inflammatory drugs (e.g. ibuprofen, mefenamic acid), hormone therapies and surgery, but these often do not give sufficient pain relief or have intolerable side effects (e.g. menopause-like symptoms with severe hot flushes, night sweats and anxiety). As a result, many women stop treatment and look for other ways to relieve their symptoms.

Cannabinoid receptors have now been identified within endometriosis lesions. Taking medical marijuana or CBD extracts may therefore help to reduce the pain and inflammation that are the hallmarks of endometriosis.

What the research shows

A national online survey of 484 Australian women with endometriosis found the most common self-help approaches included heat, rest, meditation, breathing exercises, dietary choices (such as going gluten free or vegan) and using medical marijuana or CBD. Of these, medical marijuana was the most effective (scoring an average of 7.6 out of ten) while CBD was rated almost as high (6.3 out of ten).

Over half (56%) of the women surveyed who used medical marijuana said it allowed them to reduce their other endometriosis medication by more than 50%, while a third of women using CBD were able to do the same.[38]

The most common side effects of medical marijuana were

drowsiness, increased anxiety and rapid heartbeat, whereas taking CBD was not associated with any side effects.

If you have endometriosis or period pains, it is certainly worth trying CBD to help reduce your pain, if your doctor agrees.

There is a new 'craze' for using cannabis oil-infused tampons (which melt like a pessary). I've even been asked about adding CBD oil to a normal tampon during a period. I do NOT recommend this as it could alter vaginal pH and bacterial balance, increasing the risk of toxic shock syndrome (TSS) – see page 111.

Tampons should never be used outside of a period.

Joint pain

Arthritis is the term used to describe any inflammation of the joints that causes varying degrees of pain, swelling, stiffness and reduced ability to get around.

There are many different types of arthritis, of which osteoarthritis is the most common. Other forms of arthritis can result when immune cells wrongly identify parts of a joint as 'foreign' and start to attack them. Examples of these autoimmune joint diseases include rheumatoid arthritis, ankylosing spondylitis and psoriatic arthritis (which occurs in some people with psoriasis).

Osteoarthritis is one of the most common reasons for taking CBD supplements, to help reduce the joint pain, stiffness and swelling caused by inflammation. Osteoarthritis develops when the cartilage that covers and protects bones within a joint starts to crack and flake away. The underlying bone also becomes mildly inflamed and, as the damage progresses, bones may rub together, increasing nerve irritation, pain and stiffness.

Walking awkwardly in order to ease pain in affected joints can cause ligaments and muscles to ache, and joint pain often keeps you awake at night. While osteoarthritis usually affects the larger, weight-bearing joints such as the hips, knees and lower spine, it can also affect other mobile joints such as the neck, shoulders, elbows, wrists, ankles, fingers, toes and jaw, too.

While traditionally thought of as a wear-and-tear disease, osteoarthritis is now viewed as an active process associated with inflammation and the faulty repair of damaged cartilage. Some research suggests that the endocannabinoid system is involved in regulating joint repair and protecting against osteoarthritis. Mice that lack CB2 receptors, for example, were found to experience a more rapid and severe form of osteoarthritis as they grew older compared with normal mice.[39]

What the research shows

Several studies involving human cartilage removed during total knee replacement operations or, sometimes, elderly dogs with osteoarthritis show that CBD has several different and powerful anti-arthritis actions. Among other findings, CBD appears to help suppress overactive immune cells within joints, reduces the amount of inflammatory chemicals they release and helps to stop the joint damage they cause. When dogs with osteoarthritis were treated with CBD oil or placebo, for example, both owners and vets reported a significant decrease in the pets' pain and increased activity levels in the dogs receiving CBD.

Cannabinoid receptors (CB1 and CB2) are present throughout our joints, in cartilage cells, in the synovial membrane that lines joints and within the underlying bone. CB2 receptors have also been identified in peripheral nerves within joints which might directly affect the sensitivity of joint pain receptors.

The endocannabinoids anandamide and 2-AG have also been detected in the joint lubricating oil (synovial fluid) of patients with osteoarthritis but not in those without joint symptoms. At the same time, blood levels of the endo-cannabinoid 2-AG increase as knee pain increases, and researchers believe that we make more endocannabinoids in an attempt to help reduce joint damage. There may come a time when our endocannabinoid system fails to keep up and increasing pain may reflect an endocannabinoid deficiency, although this is not yet proven. If this is the case, however, it would help to explain why taking a CBD supplement or rubbing in a CBD topical salve can not only reduce joint pain but also reduce joint swelling and inflammation.

Given that joint pain is one of the most common reasons for using CBD supplements, and that surveys show people find it effective, it is surprising that so little clinical research has actually involved people with osteoarthritis. This lack of evidence is a direct result of the restrictive legal status of cannabis plants.

Randomised placebo-controlled studies are now being planned but, in the meantime, the only way to know if CBD supplements will relieve your own joint symptoms is to try them, if your doctor agrees.

In October 2019, the US-based Arthritis Foundation issued guidance on using CBD to treat joint pain in adults, recognising the fact that arthritis is among the most common reasons for taking CBD. Their key findings, in summary, were:

- CBD may help arthritis-related pain, insomnia and anxiety, but this has not yet been confirmed in clinical trials
- There are no major safety concerns with taking CBD in moderate doses, but potential drug interactions can occur
- Never use CBD in place of the drugs prescribed to prevent permanent joint damage in inflammatory conditions such as rheumatoid arthritis (DMARDs)
- Discuss CBD with your doctor in advance and arrange follow-up evaluations every three months as is usual with any new treatment
- Start with a low dose and increase in small increments on a weekly basis if needed
- Buy CBD from a reputable company that independently tests each batch for purity, potency and safety and provides a certificate of analysis

---

Perfect Partners
If CBD alone does not improve your joint pain as much as you would like, consider adding in turmeric (you can buy combination supplements). A four-week study involving

367 people with osteoarthritis in the knee[40] found that taking turmeric extracts (1,500mg/day) was as effective as ibuprofen (1,200mg/day) for reducing pain. Those taking ibuprofen were more likely to experience side effects of abdominal pain and discomfort, however.

Neuropathic pain

Neuropathic pain is caused when a nerve is injured or irritated. This damage generates unpleasant sensations that may feel like an electric shock with burning, tingling, itching, prickling or pins and needles. Nerve damage can also cause shooting or stabbing pains or odd feelings of numbness.

A damaged nerve may trigger pain in response to a light touch, for example, or as an oversensitive response to a pinch which you would normally expect to be painful but not excruciating. While these symptoms sound similar to those that occur in fibromyalgia, the cause is different – fibromyalgia is thought to result from faulty pain perception in the brain, while neuropathic pain is caused by damage to a nerve itself. You can even feel neuropathic pain in an area that is otherwise numb or even missing (phantom limb pain).

Neuropathic pain can affect nerves anywhere in the body as a result of diabetic damage, shingles, a blood vessel pressing on its root, after an operation, due to cancer and some forms of chemotherapy, or by direct injury such as can occur in contact sports. It can also develop within the central nervous system after a stroke, spinal cord injury or a neurological condition such as multiple sclerosis.

Neuropathic pain is believed to affect one in twelve people overall. It is especially common among those with long-standing diabetes, as raised glucose levels can damage nerves.

Chronic neuropathic pain is also common following surgery due to the way that nerves are cut and cauterised, or trapped by scar tissue. According to one research study, the chance of developing long-term nerve pain after an operation is approximately 30%, and is most common following a hernia repair, open-chest surgery, mastectomy and limb amputation.[41]

Some countries, such as Canada, allow the use of medical marijuana and the pharmaceutical cannabinoid drug, nabiximols (which contains THC and CBD, see page 49) to treat neuropathic pain. In the UK, medical marijuana recently became available on private prescription from specialist clinics to treat neuropathic pain, but nabiximols (a pharmaceutical blend of cannabinoids) is not currently licensed for this use.

However, neuropathic pain is a condition for which CBD alone may help, as the number of CB2 cannabinoid receptors (with which CBD interacts) increases within the spinal cord in response to a peripheral nerve injury.[42] CBD may therefore help to suppress neuropathic pain which is often difficult to treat with conventional painkillers.

Treating neuropathic pain is challenging because of its many different causes and symptoms. As well as standard analgesics and strong opiates, antidepressants may be prescribed to boost levels of brain chemicals (neurotransmitters) that are often depleted by chronic pain. In some cases, anticonvulsant drugs are also used to help damp down overactive nerves involved in sensing pain.

In a European survey of 4,839 people with chronic pain, 64% said their prescribed painkillers were inadequate. As a result of this ineffectiveness, 48% of those with chronic pain who started taking pain medication were no longer taking them, and one in seven had stopped because of side effects.[43]

Many people with neuropathic pain who try medical marijuana find it helpful. Medical guidelines in some countries are also starting to embrace its use. In 2015, for example, the Canadian Pain Society updated their recommendations for doctors who treat neuropathic pain by moving cannabis up the list of recommended options to the third level of treatment to try if other drugs such as antidepressants and opiate painkillers have failed.

What the research shows

There is good evidence from studies involving 2,270 people that pharmaceutical cannabinoid drugs and medical marijuana can reduce neuropathic pain by between 23 and 59%. However, this comes at the cost of psychoactive effects due to the THC present in marijuana.[44]

A recent study published in the *Journal of Palliative Medicine* looked at the optimal ratio between THC and CBD for treating neuropathic pain, with the aim of helping doctors to prescribe the lowest possible amount of THC to reduce unnecessary side effects.[45]

Overall, medical marijuana (cannabis) reduced pain severity by 42%, and its effectiveness increased as the THC to CBD ratio increased. Treatment produced effective pain relief (at least a three-point reduction in pain score, see page 141) for around 20% of people using pure CBD, 40% of those using an equal blend of CBD and THC and 50% using pure THC.

This finding, that increasing levels of THC were more effective for neuropathic pain, was unexpected. Even so, it does suggest that using CBD alone is worth trying if you are not eligible for medically prescribed cannabinoid drugs or if you are unable to tolerate the side effects associated with THC.

There are currently no other clinical human studies involving CBD supplements for neuropathic pain. However, there are preclinical studies which show that CBD can suppress neuropathic pain that can occur with diabetes, cancer chemotherapy, sciatic nerve injury and spinal cord injury.

Always talk to your doctor first, and check for any interactions with your medicines before using CBD.

Cancer pain

According to the World Health Organization (WHO), an estimated 18.1 million people are newly diagnosed with cancer every year. Of these, seven out of ten people will experience pain at some point, due to direct damage by invading cancer cells or as a result of chemotherapy and radiotherapy treatments.

As pain is so common, the WHO have developed a three-step cancer 'pain ladder', which starts with non-opiate painkillers such as aspirin and paracetamol. If these are ineffective, the next step is to take a mild opiate such as codeine and finally strong opiates such as morphine. Additional medicines, such as antidepressants and anticonvulsants, are also used if necessary to help treat neuropathic pain (see page 173).

Medical marijuana is not specifically included in the WHO's pain ladder, but in countries where its use is now legal, it is increasingly recommended by cancer specialists to treat pain that is not responding to standard treatments. It is also used to suppress nausea and to stimulate a lost appetite.

Medical marijuana and cancer pain

In Israel, the Ministry of Health approved the use of medical marijuana to treat cancer pain and nausea in 2007, and this is now the most common reason for its use. A survey of almost 3,000 people using medical marijuana for cancer (prescribed as an oil, flowers, capsules or cigarettes) found that 78% said it helped them sleep, 77% said it helped their pain and 72% that it helped overcome weakness, while 65% also took it for nausea and 49% for lack of appetite. After six months, a follow-up survey found that almost all patients (95.9%) reported an improvement in their condition. The researchers concluded that medical marijuana was a well-tolerated, effective and safe option to help patients cope with their cancer-related symptoms.[46]

In the UK, a clinical study compared the effects of the pharmaceutical cannabinoid drug nabiximols against a pure

THC extract and a placebo in people with advanced cancer pain that was not improved by morphine. After two weeks' treatment, twice as many people taking the THC plus CBD blend reported a significant improvement, but pure THC did not work any better than placebo. This suggests that CBD is an important part of the treatment. It's a shame that CBD alone was not tested at the same time. Some people experienced nausea and vomiting with the THC plus CBD combination but most drug-related side effects were classed as mild to moderate.[47] In a follow-up study, it did not become less effective for relieving cancer-related pain when used long term.[48]

Unfortunately, there are currently no clinical trials assessing the effects of using CBD without THC in people with cancer pain. If you decide to try CBD, always talk to your doctor first to check that it will not interfere with your other treatments.

At present, not enough is known about how CBD affects anti-cancer drugs to provide any firm conclusions about its effectiveness and safety when used alongside them.

Only your own doctors can advise whether or not CBD may help or hinder your current treatment.

It is illegal for non-medical practitioners to make claims about treating or curing cancer with alternative treatments such as medical cannabis or CBD.

Cardiovascular health

The cardiovascular system consists of the heart and blood vessels. As we get older, our arteries tend to become less elastic and, in some cases, become narrowed due to a build-up of fatty cholesterol deposits known as plaque. This leads to common conditions such as rising blood pressure and reduced blood flow that increase the chances of having a heart attack or stroke. Contrary to popular belief, these cardiovascular conditions are not an inevitable result of ageing, however.

Recent studies suggest that our endocannabinoid system is important for maintaining a healthy heart and circulation. Anandamide helps to maintain a normal blood pressure by relaxing the artery walls, for example, and may also reduce the accumulation of cholesterol in the arteries. When oxygen levels are low, our natural endocannabinoids also help heart muscle cells to survive and prevent abnormal heart rhythms.

It has even been suggested that faulty functioning of the endocannabinoid system might be an underlying cause of cardiovascular diseases such as high blood pressure (hypertension), hardening and furring up of the arteries (atherosclerosis), heart attack, heart failure and stroke.

In laboratory studies, CBD reduced heart muscle cell damage when oxygen levels were low by 66%.[49]

High blood pressure

We need a certain pressure in our circulation to keep blood flowing round the body. This pressure depends on the pumping power of our heart, the volume of blood in our circulation, the elasticity of our blood vessels and their ability to dilate. These are all affected by various hormones, the sensitivity of special blood pressure receptors within our artery walls, how well our kidneys flush away excess sodium, diet and lifestyle factors, as well as our emotional state. For example, anger and stress cause blood pressure to increase, while feeling calm and relaxed can help it to come down.

When your blood pressure is measured, two readings are taken: the higher reading is the pressure created as your heart contracts. The lower reading is the background pressure in your circulation as your heart rests between beats.

An ideal blood pressure is one that is below 120/80 mmHg. If your blood pressure is consistently greater than this – even when you sleep – then your doctor may diagnose you as having an elevated blood pressure. If your blood pressure is above 130/80 mmHg you are diagnosed as having high blood pressure (hypertension) in the United States. In Europe, the cut-off for diagnosing hypertension is currently 140/90 mmHg, although this may change in the future.

One of the main causes of hypertension is the hardening and furring up of arteries. Known as atherosclerosis, this reduces the elasticity of your arteries so they no longer absorb the 'shock' as your heart pumps blood out into your circulation. Atherosclerosis naturally occurs with increasing age and comes on more quickly if you smoke cigarettes, drink too much alcohol, are physically unfit and follow an unhealthy diet containing too much salt and not enough fruit and vegetables. High blood pressure also runs in some families so, if your parents, brother or sister have a raised blood pressure, it's important to have yours checked regularly, too. Other causes of high blood pressure include kidney problems and some hormone imbalances.

Overall, at least one in four adults worldwide has hypertension, although not everyone is aware they have it as it causes few, if any, symptoms. If symptoms do occur, they tend to be non-specific, such as headache, nose bleeds or getting up at night to go to the toilet more often than usual.

If you haven't had your blood pressure checked in the last year, it is a good idea to do so after the age of forty. Blood pressure naturally tends to creep up with age as our arteries become less elastic.

If your blood pressure remains high and is not properly controlled (for example, by making diet and lifestyle changes and taking medication), the raised pressure will damage your arteries. In the long term, this will increase your risk of developing serious complications such as angina (heart pain), heart attack, heart failure, stroke, aortic aneurysm, peripheral vascular disease, erectile dysfunction (impotence), kidney failure and failing eyesight.

Not everyone who has raised blood pressure will need

to take antihypertensive medication immediately – most people are given an opportunity to bring down their readings by changing their diet and lifestyle.

Typical diet and lifestyle advice if you have a raised blood pressure reading:

- Stop smoking
- Lose any excess weight
- Follow a Mediterranean-style DASH (Dietary Approaches to Stop Hypertension) diet
- Cut back on your sodium/salt intake
- Increase potassium in your diet by eating more fruit and vegetables
- Exercise regularly – ideally every day
- Limit your alcohol intake
- Avoid excessive stress

There's lots of information on diet and lifestyle changes that can help lower blood pressure on my website MyLowerBloodPressure.com.

This is where CBD supplements fit in, as they may help to both prevent and treat high blood pressure by relaxing blood vessel walls and reducing anxiety and stress (which can also make your blood pressure rise).

If you are taking antihypertensive drugs or any other prescribed medicines, talk to your doctor before taking CBD supplements, and check they don't interfere with your treatment.

What the research shows

The way in which CBD lowers blood pressure may not involve the traditional cannabinoid receptors (CB1 and CB2), as its ability to lower blood pressure is also seen in animals which lack these receptors. Researchers therefore suspected there might be a previously unknown cannabinoid receptor within blood vessel walls, which they have tentatively called the endothelial cannabinoid receptor, or eCB.[50] Whether or not these eCB receptors exist remains to be seen as they have proved elusive for at least twenty years. It is now thought more likely that CBD lowers blood pressure by promoting the release of a substance called nitric oxide, which has a powerful relaxing effect on artery walls.

Nitric oxide (NO) is a gas that is naturally made in the body in tiny amounts to dilate blood vessels, lower blood pressure and increase blood flow.

Although research is in its early stages, one small clinical study involving nine men shows that CBD supplements can reduce the rise in blood pressure due to mental stress (calculating rapid arithmetic sums for two minutes), exercise stress (gripping a hand device really hard for two minutes) and cold stress (immersing a foot up to the ankle in ice slush for two minutes).[51]

When taking CBD, their systolic blood pressure (upper reading) during stress was, on average, 6 mmHg lower than when taking a placebo. The researchers believe these results were due to the anti-anxiety and painkilling effects of cannabidiol, although it may also have direct, beneficial effects on the circulation by relaxing blood vessels.

Further research is needed to confirm whether or not CBD can help to prevent or treat a raised blood pressure, however.

Cholesterol

Cholesterol is a waxy substance that is mostly made in the liver and released into the bloodstream. Although cholesterol has a bad reputation, a certain amount of it is vital for our health as cells use it to make hormones, vitamin D, bile acids and to help maintain healthy, stable, membranes that do not become too stiff.

If your cholesterol is high, however, it can contribute to hardening and furring up of the arteries. This is especially likely if you do not eat enough fruit and vegetables – these provide antioxidants that protect cholesterol within the bloodstream from oxidation. It is mainly oxidised cholesterol that builds up in artery walls to form thickenings known as plaque.

Good and bad cholesterol

We often hear about 'good cholesterol' and 'bad cholesterol' and this is because we make different types of cholesterol particle in our body. As cholesterol is insoluble, it is transported within the bloodstream by special carriers known as lipoproteins. These lipoproteins are also made in the liver and come in a variety of types. Cholesterol carried by high-density lipoproteins is known as HDL-cholesterol, and this is referred to as 'good' as its particles are too large to seep into artery walls. It also helps to mop up the 'bad' forms of cholesterol, removing them from the bloodstream and taking them back to the liver for recycling. As a result, the higher your blood level of HDL-cholesterol, the lower your risk of heart disease and stroke – an ideal HDL-cholesterol level is above 1 mmol/L for men and above 1.2 mmol/L for women.

All other forms of cholesterol (collectively known as non-HDL-cholesterol) are considered 'bad' because they are small enough to contribute to hardening and furring up of the arteries. The best known of these is low-density lipoprotein, or LDL-cholesterol.

There is some debate about the optimum blood level of the different types of 'bad' cholesterol to aim for. In general, however, an ideal total cholesterol is 5 mmol/L or less, your LDL-cholesterol should be no more than 3 mmol/L and your overall non-HDL-cholesterol no more than 4 mmol/L. Some people with a particularly high risk of having a heart attack or stroke may be set even stricter goals.

If your cholesterol levels are raised, or if you have a high risk of cardiovascular disease (even if your cholesterol isn't raised), your doctor will prescribe a drug known as a statin. Statins reduce cholesterol production in the liver and are believed to reduce the risk of a heart attack or stroke. Your doctor will also recommend diet and lifestyle changes, such as exercising more, following a Mediterranean-style diet and cutting back on fatty and processed foods, which can also improve your cholesterol balance.

If your doctor has prescribed a statin to lower your cholesterol, do not use CBD as the combination can affect your
liver. If in doubt, check with your doctor or pharmacist.

Some websites promote using CBD to lower cholesterol,
which is why it is included here. While there are some interesting laboratory studies, however, there is not yet enough
evidence to confirm that it does indeed lower cholesterol.

One study that is often quoted as evidence is a paper published in April 2011. This is said to show that taking CBD
oil can reduce the absorption of cholesterol from the diet
(where it is found in animal-derived foods such as meats,
shellfish and liver). When you actually look at the study,
however, it relates to fruit flies which were fed on hemp
seed![52] We need a lot more evidence than that on which to
base a decision to take CBD for cholesterol benefits.

What the research shows

Antioxidants are important for reducing the build-up of
cholesterol in artery walls. Latest evidence shows that CBD is
a more powerful antioxidant than either vitamin C or vitamin E. This suggests that it could well have benefits against
hardening and furring up of the arteries, but human trials
are needed to confirm this.

Research is still in its early stages and, so far, cell studies
have only looked at how CBD affects the enzymes involved
in making cholesterol. These suggest that CBD may reduce
the formation of cholesterol in artery cells, but what this

means for cholesterol levels and hardening and furring up of the arteries in real life is unclear. Also, the way CBD affects the balance between the 'good' and 'bad' forms of cholesterol is unknown.

So, while CBD *may* have beneficial effects against the consequences of 'bad' cholesterol and hardening and furring up of the arteries, this cannot be relied upon based on current evidence. If you have high cholesterol and are unwilling or unable to take statin medication (in addition to diet and lifestyle changes) and are taking CBD for another reason, it is a good idea to monitor how your cholesterol balance responds. This is easily done by a simple blood test that is available from your doctor or from some high-street pharmacies. Make sure the test provides the breakdown of your HDL-cholesterol and LDL-cholesterol levels (or, alternatively, non-HDL-cholesterol) as well as your total cholesterol.

CBD and diabetes

According to the International Diabetes Federation in 2017, an estimated 425 million adults are living with diabetes worldwide and this is expected to increase to 629 million by 2045 – largely due to the increasing rates of obesity.

The Diabetes Epidemic

An estimated 3.5 million people in the UK have a diagnosis of diabetes and an additional 549,000 have it but remain unaware of their condition. Together, this represents 6% of the UK population. According to the Centers for Disease Control and Prevention (CDC), 30.3 million people in the United States have diabetes – this represents 9.6% of the population. Another 84.1 million have pre-diabetes (poor glucose tolerance).

At least 1.2 million Australian adults (4.9% of the population) have diabetes. Over 240,000 people in New Zealand have diabetes – approximately 6% of the population. An additional 100,000 people are thought to have diabetes but are not yet diagnosed.

Glucose (a sugar) is an important fuel for all cells in the body. To avoid cells becoming overwhelmed by too much glucose, however, it can only enter muscle and fat cells through special gates (pores) that are normally closed. These gates only open when the hormone, insulin, is present. Insulin is made in the pancreas and released into the bloodstream whenever glucose levels rise above a certain level. If the pancreas stops making insulin, or if cells stop responding to insulin, then glucose is unable to enter muscle and fat cells and instead builds up in the bloodstream, causing diabetes.

There are two main types of diabetes. Type 1 diabetes occurs when immune cells start to attack and destroy the insulin-producing cells so that insulin production stops. Why this happens is unknown, but probably results from a combination of inheriting certain genes and an infection with an as-yet unidentified virus. The symptoms of untreated type 1 diabetes include fatigue, rapid weight loss, blurred vision, passing lots of urine and excessive thirst. This form of diabetes tends to affect people under the age of forty and the treatment involves insulin injections to replace the hormone no longer made in the pancreas. Type 1 diabetes cannot currently be reversed or 'cured'.

Type 2 diabetes is different, in that the pancreas continues to make some insulin, but body cells stop responding to it – a condition known as insulin resistance. Initially, the pancreas may even release more insulin in an attempt to lower blood glucose levels so that insulin levels may be higher than normal in people with type 2 diabetes, at least in the early stages of the disease. Eventually, the pancreas may become 'exhausted' so that insulin production falls. The symptoms of type 2 diabetes (such as tiredness, thirst and excess urine) develop more slowly than with type 1 diabetes and are usually less severe. Type 2 diabetes is often only diagnosed during routine medical tests or when someone develops recurrent urinary infections, thrush or boils (which are encouraged by the presence of excess glucose).

Type 2 diabetes mostly affects people over the age of forty, and is especially common in people who are very overweight or obese. Treatment involves making diet and lifestyle changes to lose weight – this can often reverse type 2 diabetes and return glucose levels back to normal, especially in the early stages of the disease. If diet and lifestyle approaches don't work, then oral drugs are prescribed to increase insulin production in the pancreas and help cells respond better to insulin. Sometimes insulin injections are also needed.

Diabetes and the endocannabinoid system

There is increasing evidence from laboratory studies that an overactive endocannabinoid system is involved in the development of diabetes and in the progression of diabetes complications (such as damage to the eyes, kidneys and nerves) that are caused by raised glucose levels, as described later. In the case of type 2 diabetes, for example, over-stimulation of CB1 cannabinoid receptors is believed to increase appetite (so you eat more and put on more weight). In the case of type 1 diabetes, a faulty endocannabinoid system may not be able to prevent immune cells from attacking the pancreas cells that make insulin, or to damp down the inflammation that makes diabetes complications worse.

CBD and Diabetes

If you have type 2 diabetes and are managing it with diet and lifestyle changes, CBD supplements may help as described below.

If you are taking any medication for type 1 or type 2 diabetes (or other health problems), it is important to talk to your doctor before taking CBD (or any other supplement) in case it interacts with your treatment. You will also need to monitor your glucose levels carefully as your doctor may need to adjust your medication if your glucose control improves (or, indeed, if it worsens).

Studies involving human cells show that cannabinoid receptors are present in the pancreas, including the cells that make insulin. Stimulating CB1 cannabinoid receptors in these cells was found to enhance insulin release, while stimulating CB2 receptors was found to lower insulin release.[53] This suggests that the endocannabinoid system is closely involved in normal glucose control.

Having a raised blood glucose level also appears to overstimulate the endocannabinoid system, so that a vicious cycle sets up and glucose control worsens.

The beneficial effects of CBD on diabetes

Although much of the research is still preclinical (which means it involves animal and cell studies rather than humans) there is growing evidence that CBD offers some benefits for people with either form of diabetes.

Even though CBD has only limited effects on CB1 and CB2 receptors on its own, it interacts with the endocannabinoid system to reduce their overactivity. It is also a powerful antioxidant that suppresses inflammation and protects struggling cells so they are more likely to survive. This might protect the pancreatic cells that secrete insulin and reduce the blood vessel and organ damage that leads to diabetes complications. It has even been suggested that CBD may protect pancreatic cells from dying in the early stages of type 1 diabetes, although this is far from proven. Researchers have found, however, that CBD lowered the risk of developing diabetes in mice who are genetically prone to diabetes.[54]

CBD and diabetes complications

If diabetes is not diagnosed and treated, high levels of glucose in the bloodstream will damage the arteries so they are more likely to harden and fur up (atherosclerosis). This increases the risk of developing high blood pressure, impotence, heart disease and stroke. Raised glucose levels also damage our internal organs and nerves, and diabetes is a leading cause of loss of vision, kidney failure and painful nerve damage (neuropathy, see page 173). If you have diabetes, it is therefore important to ensure that your glucose levels remain well controlled by following your doctor's advice about diet and lifestyle, and taking any medication you are prescribed.

Some of these complications of diabetes are due to the excess production of a damaging substance (sorbitol) inside cells. This substance is made from glucose by the action of a particular enzyme (aldose reductase) and researchers hope to develop new drugs that block this enzyme in order to prevent diabetes complications. CBD was recently found to reduce the activity of this enzyme by more than 70%, making it a strong contender as a potentially protective supplement for people with diabetes.[55]

CBD and heart disease in diabetes
Heart muscle cells contain cannabinoid receptors and laboratory studies suggest that CBD may help to protect these cells when their blood supply is reduced as a result of diabetes. Other studies have found that CBD helps to improve energy production in heart muscle cells.[57] This may explain why CBD helped them to survive and reduced the formation of scar tissue in mice with diabetic heart damage.[58]

CBD also has powerful antioxidant (see page 65) and anti-inflammatory effects and researchers believe that CBD may help to protect against atherosclerosis, coronary artery disease and other diabetes complications.

CBD and kidney disease in diabetes

Diabetes is one of the main causes of kidney failure and this complication has been linked with overactivity of CB1 cannabinoid receptors. As CBD helps to reduce the overstimulation of CB1 receptors, it may help to reduce the kidney damage caused by high glucose levels.

CBD and eye disease in diabetes

Diabetes is a leading cause of blindness as high blood glucose levels cause blood vessels in the retina to leak and damage light-sensitive cells. This complication is known as diabetic retinopathy. In people with diabetic eye disease, the number of CB1 cannabinoid receptors in the eye increases. Blocking these CB1 receptors was found to protect human retina cells from damage, and to help prevent retinal damage in diabetic mice.[59] It is believed, therefore, that CBD may have a role in protecting against eye complications caused by diabetes.

CBD and nerve disease in diabetes

Persistently raised glucose levels damage nerves and can lead to burning or stabbing pain, electric sensations and numbness (neuropathy, see page 173). Known as diabetic neuropathy, these symptoms eventually affect as many as two out of three people with diabetes. Research suggests that CBD may help to slow the progression of diabetic nerve damage by blocking the overstimulation of CB1 receptors.[60] This has not yet been researched in humans, however.

CBD and insulin resistance

Overactivity of the endocannabinoid system is increasingly thought to be a root cause of obesity and insulin resistance in type 2 diabetes. Overstimulation of CB1 receptors in the brain can increase appetite and food intake, for example, and blocking these receptors helps to decrease hunger and reduce food cravings. CB1 receptors in the liver and fat cells also help to regulate the production and storage of fats, and where this fat is stored – especially around the waist. By blocking CB1 receptors, CBD may help to support weight loss as well as improving insulin resistance, although this is still under investigation.

*

As a result of all these studies, and the excellent safety and tolerability of CBD, researchers strongly believe that it has great therapeutic potential in treating diabetic complications. Good quality human studies are needed to confirm this, however. So, don't start taking CBD without discussing it with your doctor first.

CBD and weight loss

CBD is gaining a reputation as an effective weight-loss supplement. This may seem surprising given that marijuana is associated with the munchies! This is because THC in marijuana stimulates CB1 receptors, which not only triggers hunger but also appears to make food smell more enticing by increasing your sensitivity to smells.

The endocannabinoid system first appeared millions of years ago within the animal kingdom to control feeding responses and opening and closing of the mouth when food is detected.

Overstimulation of CB1 receptors by our own endocannabinoids (anandamide and 2-AG) may contribute to obesity by increasing the desire for snacking as well as the amount of fat you store. By blocking this overstimulation, CBD may help to reduce hunger signals and promote fat burning rather than fat storage.

BAT versus WAT

The fat stored under your skin comes in two main types: white adipose tissue (WAT) which *stores* fat, and brown adipose tissue (BAT) which *burns* fat.

Brown fat is what keeps hibernating animals alive during their winter sleep and, in humans, helps infants to stay warm while they are too small to generate heat by shivering. As we get older, however, our fat-burning BAT fat slowly disappears. The lucky few who retain a good amount of BAT continue to burn more fat to generate heat and are less likely to put on weight. Those who lose most of their BAT fat tend to put on weight more easily and are more likely to develop type 2 diabetes.

In an exciting finding, scientists have discovered that some white fat cells continue to show a few brown-like characteristics, dubbing this 'beige' fat.[61] What's more, researchers believe there is a way to convert this beige fat into brown fat to help overweight people lose weight.[62] The race is on to find a drug to do just that, but in the meantime it seems that CBD can help, too.

CBD promotes fat burning

In laboratory studies, CBD causes white fat cells to act more like they are brown and burn more fat. It does this by switching on eight genes that are normally only active in brown fat and, at the same time, reduces the activity of three genes involved in fat storage. This makes CBD a potentially promising treatment in the war against obesity.[63]

Another recent finding is that CBD binds to a receptor (TPRV-1) which helps to regulate body temperature. This may stimulate fat burning to maintain a higher body temperature.

Other ways in which CBD may help you lose weight include effects on brain neurotransmitters, such as serotonin, which help to regulate our appetite; by reducing anxiety (which can lead to comfort eating) and effects on gut bacteria which are now also thought to affect our appetite (see page 151).

Although CBD has been identified as a potential anti-obesity treatment, however, clinical trials are needed to confirm this.

The sad tale of Rimonabant
Rimonabant was a synthetic cannabinoid drug that was launched in over fifty countries in 2006 as a

prescription-only treatment for obesity. Rimonabant blocked CB1 cannabinoid receptors to reduce appetite. In clinical trials, one in three obese people taking rimonabant lost 10% of their body weight and kept their weight down for two years. Unfortunately, however, rimonabant was withdrawn in 2008 because of reported side effects of anxiety and depression.[64] Importantly, CBD has not been associated with these side effects.

CBD and herpes virus infections

Herpes simplex is the virus that causes cold sores. There are two variations, types 1 and 2, of which herpes simplex virus type 1 is the most common. According to the World Health Organization, as many as 3.7 billion people under the age of fifty (two thirds of the population) are infected with herpes simplex virus type 1, and another 417 million are infected with herpes simplex virus type 2.

Herpes viruses are passed on through close contact. The initial, or primary, infection often passes unnoticed or may only produce mild soreness if you have a good natural immunity against the virus. Occasionally, however, herpes viruses cause excruciatingly painful sores around the mouth or genitals.

Herpes simplex virus type 1 is the main cause of oral cold sores, but can also cause genital herpes. Herpes simplex virus type 2 is the main cause of genital herpes but can also cause oral cold sores.

Herpes is a lifelong infection as, during the first attack, swarms of viral particles travel up nerve endings and lie dormant in a swelling (ganglion) near the nerve root. When your immunity is suppressed, these viruses can reactivate and travel down the nerve to cause a recurrence. A recurrence may occur weeks, months or even years after the initial infection. Some people have few, if any, recurrences, but around one in three people who carry these viruses experience regular outbreaks.

Common triggers for herpes recurrences include physical and emotional stress, other infections (e.g. a common cold) and exposure to ultraviolet light (e.g. sunbeds, skiing holidays).

When herpes viruses reactivate and travel back down a nerve, they often produce characteristic tingling, burning, itching or lightening pains, which are known as a prodrome. These symptoms last for twelve to twenty-four hours and usually herald the appearance of one or more blisters. The blisters develop once viral particles reach the skin, spreading from cell to cell and hijacking their nucleus to make more viruses. This kills the cells, releasing new viruses and creating a blister that bursts to form a shallow ulcer. These ulcers are particularly painful as the underlying nerve endings are exposed. Eventually, the ulcers crust and scab over to heal within ten to fourteen days and the cycle starts over again as new viruses travel up to the nerve ganglion to lie dormant.

CBD is a potentially effective treatment to suppress cold sore recurrences caused by herpes simplex viruses. The immune cells that fight viral infections have numerous CB1 and CB2 receptors, as have the nerves in which herpes viruses lie hidden until such times as they reactivate.

The endocannabinoid system may influence whether or not you are troubled with frequent herpes recurrences. Overstimulation of CB1 receptors (by our own endocannabinoids, or by the THC in marijuana) appears to increase the chance of a recurrence, while the CB2 receptors found on immune cells (with which CBD interacts) appear to help suppress recurrences.

Research is still in its early stages, but this has not stopped CBD being widely touted on the internet as stopping herpes outbreaks. One site states, optimistically, that thousands of studies show that CBD can positively affect herpes viruses. There are not thousands of studies, but a mere handful, most of which relate to mice and guinea pigs. So far, there are no human clinical studies to confirm that CBD suppresses herpes recurrences, but in theory it should work.

What the research shows

The first report linking cannabis with recurrent herpes was published in the *British Medical Journal* back in 1972. A doctor from the Radcliffe Infirmary in Oxford described a 30-year-old male whose frequent recurrences of genital herpes usually occurred within two or three days of smoking a 'reefer'. When he stopped smoking marijuana, the attacks became infrequent but returned when he started again. Other patients reported similar experiences.[65]

Later studies identified THC as the component within

cannabis that decreases immune resistance to herpes simplex viruses. Even low doses of THC suppressed resistance to herpes simplex type 2 infection in mice by a staggering ninety-six-fold.[66]

It's now known that THC inhibits the release of calcium in nerve cells, which can create ideal conditions for herpes viruses to reactivate. What's more, THC interferes with the effectiveness of immune cells that fight herpes simplex viruses so that using marijuana can make symptoms more severe.

In contrast, CBD acts on CB2 receptors to boost immune responses and suppress inflammation and viral infections. In laboratory cell tests, CBD even helped to suppress the effects of another type of herpes virus that causes a form of cancer (Kaposi's sarcoma), affecting blood and lymph vessels in people with severe immunosuppression.[67] This suggests that its effects against herpes viruses may be quite powerful, although it has not yet been tested in patients.

Anecdotal reports suggest that CBD is effective so, if you are experiencing troublesome outbreaks, it is worth a try. Do check for interactions with any medications you are taking, however.

A personal story
As I was writing this book, I developed the telltale itching and burning of a lip cold sore which quickly swelled to the size of a pea.

I started applying CBD oil (just 3% strength as that was all I had) and the pain diminished within five minutes. I repeated the applications every half-hour until bedtime. Next morning, the swelling was significantly reduced and remained beneath the surface without breaking through the skin.

I continued to apply the CBD oil regularly and the cold sore was gone within twenty-four hours without forming an ulcer. Although this is only a personal anecdote, I am impressed as over-the-counter creams have never worked well for me.

CBD for skin problems

During childhood, we quickly learned that 'rubbing it better' really does work for reducing the pain of any knocks and sprains. The action of rubbing stimulates the nerve endings in our skin, helping to overwhelm the pain signals reaching our brain so that we perceive less pain. This same concept plays a role when we use rub-in ointments and creams to treat sports injuries and painful muscles and joints in later life. The physical action of massaging in a topical cream or ointment also helps to warm the area, which increases blood flow, bringing in more of the oxygen, nutrients and immune factors needed for healing. When rubbing is combined with an active ingredient that is absorbed into the skin, such as CBD, the benefits are multiplied.

Cannabis poultices have been applied to wounds to stimulate healing for thousands of years. As well as having antioxidant and antiseptic properties, hemp extracts suppress pain and inflammation through direct effects on the cannabinoid receptors that are present on skin cells and the underlying nerve endings. When CBD is infused into soothing balms and applied, it helps to soothe chapped, dry or irritated skin and moisturise scars.

Endocannabinoid receptors are present on and within skin cells, skin nerve endings, skin macrophages (scavenger cells), mast cells (which release histamine – a chemical involved in allergic reactions), hair follicles, oil and sweat glands.

The skin forms an important barrier between the body and the outside world, and faulty functioning of the endocannabinoid system is thought to contribute to many different skin conditions including acne, seborrhoeic dermatitis (greasy inflammation), dryness, allergic dermatitis, eczema, psoriasis, hair growth disorders and even skin cancers.

When applied to the skin, CBD acts on local cannabinoid receptors to reduce inflammation and pain and has an antihistamine effect to relieve itching. CBD may therefore help to soothe dry, irritated or inflamed skin conditions and suppress allergic skin reactions. So it's not surprising that skincare ranges infused with CBD are already available.

Topical CBD products are used to help treat inflammatory conditions such as acne, eczema and psoriasis, and for softening scars. Medical marijuana is also used in some countries to treat psoriasis, dermatitis, pruritus (itching) and skin rashes associated with an autoimmune condition called lupus.

Some dermatologists are concerned, however, because dispensaries in Canada, Europe and the United States are starting to promote medical marijuana for treating skin conditions such as acne, wrinkles, allergic contact dermatitis, Lyme disease, discoloured blemishes and even serious skin conditions such as epidermolysis bullosa (an autoimmune condition in which the skin blisters) and melanoma (a form of skin cancer), despite the fact that there is not yet enough research to confirm the effectiveness of medical marijuana or CBD in these conditions since it has only been tested in laboratory studies rather than humans.

However, an online survey of dermatologists in the US in 2018 found that nearly all who responded (94%) believe it is worthwhile to research cannabinoids for treating skin conditions. More than half (55%) reported that at least one patient had asked them about cannabinoids in the last year and most (86%) said they would be willing to prescribe an FDA-approved cannabinoid as a topical treatment if one were available (although at the time of writing there are none).[68]

What the research shows

Cannabinoids are anti-inflammatory and our own endocannabinoid, anandamide, helps to regulate the way cells divide to avoid their overgrowth. In psoriasis, however, inflammation causes skin cells to divide up to ten times faster than normal. As a result, the new skin cells form characteristic raised, red patches covered with fine, silvery scales.

In one study, CBD, THC, CBN (cannabinol) and CBG (cannabigerol) were tested to see if they could stop this overgrowth of human psoriasis skin cells under laboratory conditions.[69] All the cannabinoids tested were able to do this, but CBD and CBG had the greatest overall activity. Interestingly, the effectiveness of CBD was not reduced by adding a substance known to block cannabinoid receptors, so how it works is a bit of a mystery if it does not work via the usual CB1 and CB2 cannabinoid receptors. Even so, this study does support a potential role for CBD in the treatment of psoriasis.

A recent small study from Italy tested a CBD ointment on twenty people with psoriasis or atopic dermatitis (eczema), some of whom also had scarring. They were asked to apply the CBD ointment to affected areas of skin twice a day for three months. During this period they did not use any other skincare products. After three months, significant improvements were noted by patients and clinicians, especially in skin hydration and elasticity. The appearance of blemishes and scarring improved and none of those taking part reported any irritation or allergic reactions to the CBD ointment. As a result, the researchers concluded that applying a topical CBD ointment is both a safe and effective way to improve the quality of life for people with troublesome skin disorders, including inflammatory conditions such as eczema and psoriasis.[70]

Another small study assessed the effects of CBD in just three people with a rare, serious skin disease called pyoderma gangrenosum, in which deep ulcers develop on the lower legs. This extremely painful condition is usually treated with powerful steroid creams that suppress inflammation (corticosteroids) plus oral and topical morphine (although there are concerns that opioids may inhibit wound healing). In this study, a medicinal cannabis oil (containing THC plus CBD) was applied to the wounds one to three times a day. Each patient reported an almost immediate relief from pain, which started within three to five minutes of each application. Their average daily level of pain also fell by between 65 and 73.4% – this is significant, given that pain reductions of more than 30% are considered a clinically meaningful result.[71]

While these studies are only small, exploratory trials, their results suggest that larger studies are warranted to confirm what applying CBD or medicinal cannabis oil can (and can't) do for a wide range of skin conditions.

Although anecdotal evidence from internet forums suggests cannabinoids may help some skin conditions such as eczema and psoriasis, don't expect a miracle cure. Larger trials are needed to compare the effects of CBD salves against a placebo before dermatologists are able to draw any definite conclusions.

Topical CBD for pain relief

Many people use an oral CBD supplement to help alleviate their pain as described earlier in this chapter. You can also use a topical CBD product in addition to your oral pain medication, which may help to reduce the number of tablets you need to control your pain. CBD acts on cannabinoid receptors in nerve fibres within the skin to help reduce pain. Interestingly, by stimulating CB2 receptors in the skin, CBD may also trigger the release of our own morphine-like painkiller, called beta-endorphin, for an additional pain-relieving effect.

When CBD gel is applied topically, some is also absorbed into the bloodstream to help reduce inflammation elsewhere in the body. It's also possible that immune cells 'primed' by CBD in the skin might travel to sites of inflammation to help reduce pain and swelling. For example, studies involving animals with arthritis show that rubbing CBD gel into a small patch of skin on the back for thirty seconds helps to reduce inflammation, swelling and pain in their arthritic knees after four days of regular treatment.[72]

As a result of this experiment, the researchers concluded that rubbing a 10% CBD gel into the skin directly overlaying an inflamed joint would help to reduce pain and inflammation alongside other treatments. This has not yet been tested in human volunteers but, if the growing sales of CBD salves is anything to go by, it appears that consumers are finding it effective.

How to use a topical CBD product

Topical CBD creams and salves are made by infusing CBD extracts into a soothing and softening emollient made from ingredients such as beeswax, shea butter and oils such as coconut, argan and rosehip. Therapeutic essential oils may be added to this, such as geranium, eucalyptus, lavender or chamomile. Other ingredients such as menthol, oil of wintergreen or capsicum (an extract from chilli peppers) are sometimes added to provide additional cooling or warming effects. Known as counterirritants, these salves provide a low-level, continuous stimulation of the nerve endings in the skin so they literally run out of signalling chemicals, become less sensitive and pass on fewer pain signals to the brain. The low level of signals that do get through tend to get screened out as they pass through special 'pain gates' in the spinal cord – this is how the body shuts off distracting irritation such as localised pain, itching, irritation or soreness.

- When using a CBD ointment or cream for the first time, apply a small amount to a clean, healthy area of skin and wait awhile to see how your skin responds to the ingredients. Don't apply a topical treatment to broken skin without testing a small area first, in case it stings
- If there is no reaction, apply a thin layer of CBD ointment or cream (sometimes called a salve or balm on the label) and massage thoroughly into the affected area of skin (or, if you have arthritis, over a painful joint)
- Ideally, apply topical CBD ointment or cream after a warm bath or shower, or after exercise, as warmth helps the skin to absorb it more quickly for a faster action
- Always follow the directions on the packaging as some CBD products may need to be used at regular intervals while others are designed to be used as and when necessary
- It may help to wear a warming joint or sports wrap (available from pharmacies) after applying the treatment. (Check the product leaflet first in case the manufacturer does not advise this)
- Avoid touching or rubbing your eyes while using the cream or ointment and always wash your hands after applying it

You can also apply CBD from a dropper bottle to your skin (this can work well when using CBD to treat a herpes lip cold sore).

7

CBD for
Emotional Wellbeing

Nurturing our mental health is just as important as looking after our physical health. When our emotions are in balance, we have an inner strength that allows us to cope better with the challenges of everyday life.

Traditionally, some people in need of emotional support have turned to marijuana for its relaxation and 'stoned' effects, which can help to blank out or numb emotional problems. Taking it over a long period of time can cause it to become less effective, however, leading to the need to take an ever higher dose to get the same effect, which can, in turn, lead to addiction.

As CBD has similar relaxation benefits but without the 'high' or 'stoned' feelings caused by THC in marijuana, it is increasingly being used instead of marijuana for its ability to produce general feelings of wellbeing.

In the sections that follow we will look at how and why so

many people find CBD useful for aiding relaxation, reducing stress and anxiety, lifting a low mood, improving sleep and quitting smoking – included here as it can cause emotional symptoms such as anxiety, irritability and cravings as well as physical symptoms such as trembling and sweating.

If you have a serious mental health condition such as psychosis, depression or post-traumatic stress, it is important not to self-medicate but to follow the advice and treatment recommended by your own doctor.

CBD and stress

Stress is a modern term first used by Dr Hans Selye, a Hungarian endocrinologist (hormone specialist) in 1936 to describe the effects of change on the body. The word is now known to us all as encapsulating the unpleasant physical and emotional symptoms associated with excess tension.

A certain amount of pressure is needed to get us out of bed in the mornings and primes us to meet life's challenges. The negative effects of stress only develop when mental pressure increases to the degree that we feel unable to cope. Where this point lies will vary from person to person, and also from time to time, as it depends on many factors including the quality of our diet, how physically fit we are, how much sleep we're getting and what else is going on in our lives and relationships. When we are overwhelmed by stress, we might feel anxious and restless, with racing thoughts, trembling muscles and sweaty palms, and be unable to sleep.

Feeling stressed simply means you are under more pressure (which may be real or perceived) than you feel comfortable with at a particular point in time.

These symptoms are due to our natural stress response, which puts our body on red alert. In ancient times, this helped our ancestors survive by preparing to react quickly to a dangerous situation. This is known as the 'fight-or-flight' response and when we are in this state our:

- blood glucose level rises to provide our muscles and brain with instant energy
- pupils dilate to widen our field of vision to help us look for danger
- bowels, bladder (and sometimes stomach) empty so we are lighter for running
- circulation to the gut shuts down and more blood is diverted to muscle
- pulse and blood pressure go up, and we breathe more deeply to increase the blood and oxygen going to our muscles and brain
- memory and ability to think straight improve
- sensitivity to pain is reduced

Nowadays, we rarely burn off these stress responses by fighting or fleeing; instead, we remain primed for a vigorous physical response that never comes. If we remain in this state for a long time – for example, because we are overworking, are not getting on with our partner, or our child is seriously ill – this elevated state of stress can lead to the taut, quivering muscles, tremor, tension, distraction and feelings of edginess that we may experience with long-term stress. We may also develop a constant sinking feeling in the pit of our stomach, become overly alert and experience excessive and undue worry.

Stress is among the most common reasons that people take CBD as, according to user surveys, they find it helps to reduce anxiety and aid relaxation. While there are currently few clinical trials investigating its effectiveness in humans, some laboratory studies provide plausible explanations for why it might work.

Stress and the endocannabinoid system

Our endocannabinoid system helps to shape how we interpret our surroundings and how we respond emotionally to changing conditions, and is closely involved in regulating our emotional, physical and behavioural responses to stress. Researchers have found that during periods of acute stress, levels of one of our endocannabinoids, anandamide, appears to drop while levels of the other main endocannabinoid, 2-AG, increase. This is believed to help us think more clearly under pressure, reduce the degree to which we feel pain, help us blank out stressful memories and bring us back to the more normal emotional and physical state. At the same time, chronic stress causes CB1 receptors to become less active or even disappear altogether in almost every region of the brain.

It's now thought that this disruption of endocannabinoid signalling plays a key role in both triggering the stress response and bringing it to a timely end. Our adrenal glands continue to release the stress hormone cortisol until our level of 2-AG rises enough to switch this off. If this system of checks and balances doesn't work properly, for example if our anandamide levels fall too low, or our 2-AG levels do not increase sufficiently, we may become more vulnerable to stress-related conditions such as anxiety, depression and post-traumatic stress. CBD is known to help increase levels of anandamide to correct them if they fall too low, which may partly account for its ability to reduce feelings of stress. If you are experiencing any of the symptoms below, then a CBD supplement (in the form of capsules, drops, oral spray or gummies) may help.

The psychological symptoms of persistent stress (i.e. stress that is not resolving as quickly as you might expect) are:

- Frustration
- Difficulty concentrating
- Muddled thinking
- A tendency to lose perspective
- Difficulty making rational judgements
- A tendency to make rash decisions
- Negative thoughts
- Loss of self-confidence
- Lost sense of humour
- Feelings of impending doom

The physical symptoms of persistent stress are:

- Sweaty palms
- Dry mouth

- Rapid pulse
- Tense muscles
- Lump in the throat
- Butterflies in the stomach
- Trembling
- Frequent visits to the bathroom
- Loose bowels
- Erratic breathing with a tendency to hyperventilate
- Panic attacks

If stress continues over a long period and becomes chronic (which different researchers define as lasting for at least one month, three months, six months or twelve months) you will feel drained of energy and are likely to experience:

- Tiredness all the time
- Insomnia and bad dreams
- Tension headaches
- Indigestion
- Nausea
- Loss of sex drive
- Sexual difficulties such as low libido or, for men, erectile difficulties
- Frequent infections due to impaired immunity

Long-term (chronic) stress can also exacerbate pre-existing conditions such as asthma, eczema, psoriasis and irritable bowel syndrome, and contribute towards potentially serious health problems such as poor glucose tolerance, diabetes, high blood pressure, stroke, angina and heart attack.

Non-competitive exercise is one of the best ways to reduce the adverse effects of stress as it helps to burn off the effects of stress hormones that have primed your body for exercise as part of the fight-or-flight response. Choose any form of exercise you enjoy, such as walking, swimming, cycling, dancing or gardening. It's best to avoid competitive exercise such as racing as this could simply add to your level of stress.

As we feel more and more stressed, we may adopt behavioural strategies that, although they may help us feel better in the short term, affect our long-term health and only serve to further undermine our ability to cope. These might include using alcohol, cigarettes and recreational drugs (including medical marijuana) to help us 'cope' and feel less stressed. We may also comfort-eat, skip meals, avoid socialising or start to act in impulsive ways in order to feel more in control. For example, there is a common saying that someone is 'tearing their hair out' when they are really stressed. This refers to an irresistible urge, or compulsion, to pull hair from the scalp, eyebrows or elsewhere (trichotillomania) which, in some cases, is used as a way to help relieve stress.

Although research is in its early stages, it is thought that some of these behavioural changes may be driven by an imbalance within the endocannabinoid system that leads to emotional responses such as cravings for food or nicotine. This might occur if stress reduces our ability to produce enough of our own endocannabinoids (anandamide and 2-AG), for example, or if the number of cannabinoid receptors with which they interact is reduced so that, over-all, the endocannabinoid system becomes less active than usual. How or why this happens is not yet known but, if this theory is correct, it provides a basis for explaining why CBD might help, as explained below.

Chocolate Cravings

When eating food for pleasure, such as chocolate, blood levels of our endocannabinoids, anandamide and 2-AG, increase. This is thought to cause the pleasurable feelings that make us want more.

When we're stressed, relaxation techniques such as meditation can help us find inner calm, but, as many of us know, relaxing is easier said than done. The pace of modern life means it's easy to lose the ability to switch off and this is where CBD can help. CBD works with our endocannabinoid system and other brain chemicals (such as serotonin and melatonin) to reduce our response to stress, damp down the overactivity in parts of the brain that occurs when we feel anxious and helps us relax. CBD also appears to reduce the oversecretion of cortisol, our main stress hormone.

When you take CBD you may notice a relaxing effect which comes on within twenty minutes to an hour, depending on how you take it (oral sprays and drops held in the mouth work more quickly than capsules). These effects can last for up to twelve hours, depending on the dose. You may also notice a pleasant and perceptible lift in your mood. Some people describe feeling a wave of calm and even bliss washing over them, although it does not produce a 'high' in the same way as the THC in marijuana does.

If you want to try CBD to help with your stress, start with a low dose (5mg to 10mg) taken two or three times a day. If necessary, slowly increase the dose every few days to find what works best for you. If, after a couple of weeks, you have not noticed a good response, despite taking the manufacturer's recommended maximum dose, then you may benefit from a different type of CBD product (a full-spectrum oil, for example, see page 94). You should also check that the product you are taking is made to pharmaceutical standards (known as GMP, see page 100) as it may contain less CBD than claimed on the label. Read chapter five for more information on how to use CBD safely.

Burn-out and adrenal fatigue

The term 'burn-out' was first used in 1974 by psychologist Herbert Freudenberger, who defined it as the extinction of motivation or incentive – in other words, losing your get-up-and-go. Burn-out (with a hyphen) is now included in the World Health Organization International Classification of Disease as a work-related issue, although it is not considered a medical condition as such.

Some people may describe themselves as 'burned out' when overwhelmed with other stressful issues in their life, but the official definition limits the term to excessive and prolonged stress at work. Essentially, it is a state of extreme emotion, with a loss of energy, exhaustion, and negative or cynical feelings, which leaves you too drained to continue doing your job effectively. You may start to feel detached and disengaged from your surroundings, friends or colleagues and may well feel empty, hopeless and helpless, with little motivation to do anything. If it continues, you can become severely depressed and life may seem like it is not worth living. If you think you are experiencing burn-out, it is essential to seek help and advice from your doctor and from your line manager or human resources department at work.

Adrenal fatigue is another term that is often used to describe the physical and emotional symptoms caused by excessive and chronic (long-term) stress. This is not a medically recognised diagnosis but is another way to describe stress-related symptoms such as widespread aches, fatigue, nervousness, sleep disturbances and digestive problems. These symptoms are traditionally said to occur when the adrenal glands have become too depleted to continue making the stress hormones needed to maintain the constant alertness of the fight-or-flight response.

These emotional and physical manifestations of burn-out and adrenal fatigue are exactly what you would expect if, instead, it was the endocannabinoid system that was depleted. They fit what would be expected to happen if you were unable to replenish your falling levels of anandamide or to sustain the raised levels of 2-AG needed to help damp down the stress response and bring it to a timely end.

And so this is where CBD comes in, as it is believed to prop up anandamide and 2-AG levels to help reset the stress response back to the more normal non-stressed mode, which is often described as 'rest-and-digest' – the opposite of the 'fight-or-flight' response.

What the research shows

While much of the research into the effects of stress on the endocannabinoid system has involved laboratory studies, some studies have now been carried out on stressed volunteers.

So far, researchers have confirmed that people with high levels of anxiety, stress or depression have lower blood levels of anandamide than those who are not anxious or stressed. Brain scans have also shown that cannabinoids damp down overactivity in a part of the brain called the amygdala, which is involved in our fear response to threatening situations, and increase blood flow to parts of the brain involved in reasoning and forming ordered thoughts (known to psychologists as cognition).[2]

Stress is not just caused by extreme emotions but also by severe physical conditions. Some evidence of how our endocannabinoids help us to adapt and overcome severe physical and emotional stress comes from a study in which twenty-one brave volunteers took part in the so-called 'vomit comet', which mimics weightlessness in space. Some people enjoy its rollercoaster-like manoeuvres, while others become severely stressed. In this study, blood levels of anandamide fell in those who were severely stressed by motion sickness while levels of 2-AG remained the same. In those who did not become stressed by motion sickness, levels of both their endocannabinoids, anandamide and 2-AG, increased. Overall, these results suggest that our susceptibility to severe physical and emotional stress (in this case due to motion sickness) may depend on how well our endocannabinoid system responds to produce more or less of each of our endocannabinoids.[3]

While more clinical evidence is needed, there is enough anecdotal evidence from user surveys to suggest that if you suffer from acute stress it's worth trying CBD to see if it alleviates your symptoms.

Post-traumatic stress disorder

Post-traumatic stress disorder (PTSD) is an increasingly common condition that can occur after someone experiences an extremely stressful and traumatic event, such as a sudden bereavement, violence or abuse. PTSD affects between one in ten and one in twenty people at some point in their life, causing upsetting memories and flashbacks of the traumatic event or events, difficulty sleeping and nightmares. The usual treatments for PTSD include cognitive behavioural therapy (CBT), in which people are encouraged to talk through their experiences with a therapist in detail, alongside antidepressants if needed. Another therapy that is sometimes recommended is EMDR (eye movement desensitisation and reprocessing), in which rapid, rhythmic eye movements are used to help dampen emotionally charged memories of past traumatic events.

It's now thought that PTSD may involve faulty responses within the endocannabinoid system, which usually helps us to process memories and suppress those that are particularly traumatic. Some studies have found that people with PTSD tend to have levels of anandamide in their blood that are, on average, half those found in people without PTSD. They also have an increased number of cannabinoid receptors, which creates a mismatch as there are too few endocannabinoids and too many receptors, leaving them under-stimulated. CBD may help to overcome this mismatch by prolonging the effects of anandamide. Another way in which it might help is by interacting with serotonin receptors which help to lift the mood.

What the research shows

The effectiveness of cannabidiol was tested in a recent small study involving eleven people with PTSD who were attending an outpatient psychiatry clinic. CBD was added to their normal medications and talking therapy for eight weeks, at a dose of 25mg once or twice a day, as needed. Ten out of the eleven people reported a reduction in their PTSD symptoms, with the severity of their symptoms falling, on average, by 28%.[4] (Do not try to do this alone without the support of your own doctor, especially if you are taking prescribed medications, as interactions might occur that could reduce the effectiveness of your medical treatment or increase the chance of unwanted side effects.)

Another study found that CBD reduced feelings of fear in volunteers who were conditioned to expect an electric shock on seeing a coloured box. Inhaling CBD after the shock helped them forget the experience and reduced their level of anxiety and fear when they saw the coloured boxes again later.[5] Larger trials are now needed to confirm these findings.

221

CBD and anxiety

Anxiety is one of the most common reasons for taking CBD, second only to pain overall. While anxiety is a natural and appropriate survival instinct in some situations, it can take over your life when it gets out of hand. According to a UK survey commissioned by the Mental Health Foundation and published in 2014, almost one in five of us feel anxious nearly all of the time or a lot of the time, and more than half of us have noticed that other people are more anxious today than they were five years ago as a result of pressure at work, home and in their social lives.

Anxiety is not a one-size-fits-all diagnosis, however, as there are several different types of anxiety and different people will experience it differently. Sometimes we just feel anxious for no identifiable reason, which is often described as 'free-floating anxiety'. At other times, our reaction to relatively minor things such as missing the bus, losing a pair of glasses or a mobile phone running out of charge can become out of all proportion due to what psychologists describe as 'fearcasting' or 'catastrophising', in which we leap ahead to all the worst-case scenarios – most of which may of course never happen. For example, you may worry that you will make a mistake at work, and that if you do so you will lose your job. You may then leap to the conclusion that you are likely to lose your job and start to worry about all the repercussions of losing it, reacting as if it is an inevitability or at least extremely likely, rather than an extreme and unlikely outcome. This, understandably, generates feelings of panic and losing control, which makes the anxiety worse. (Panic attacks are discussed in more detail below.)

The difference between chronic stress and anxiety disorders is not always easy to work out, but stress is mainly due to external pressures beyond our control that we find hard to cope with. In contrast, an anxiety disorder arises from within and the way we perceive ourselves and is linked with poor self-esteem.

It seems that women are especially prone to anxiety and are two-and-a-half times more likely to be affected than men. This is partly due to the way our neural pathways are wired, and partly because of the effects of hormonal changes at different phases of the menstrual cycle and at the menopause.

CBT (cognitive behavioural therapy) and other types of counselling are the most common treatment for all forms of anxiety and antidepressants are often also prescribed, but tranquillisers such as diazepam are avoided as much as possible as they can be addictive.

Generalised anxiety disorder (GAD) affects an estimated one in twenty of us in the UK. It is diagnosed when you have spent at least six months worrying excessively about a number of everyday problems. For example, you are always anticipating disaster and feel unable to relax because of worrying about your health, finances, family or career – or sometimes just the thought of having to get through the day. You may also experience depression, with feelings of sadness and hopelessness and loss of appetite, and you might find that you are waking up very early. The symptoms of generalised anxiety disorder include:

- Worrying excessively about ordinary situations
- An inability to control your worrying
- The fear that something awful might happen
- Feeling on edge and finding it difficult to relax and sit still
- Irritability
- Muscle tension
- Sleep disturbance

Social anxiety (which is also known as social phobia) affects around one in fourteen of us and is similar in some ways to extreme shyness. It stems from an extreme fear of being the centre of attention, or of being humiliated or embarrassed in front of others. If you have a social anxiety disorder, you are likely to think that everyone is better at socialising than you and to dread everyday activities such as meeting strangers, making conversation with people you don't know very well, speaking on the phone or just walking into a crowded room. The most common social anxiety is a fear of public speaking, but some people experience overwhelming anxiety (or phobia) about using a public toilet or eating in front of other people. People with social anxiety will go out of their way to avoid social occasions, to the point where it severely impacts on their personal life and career. The most common symptoms of social anxiety disorder (which is diagnosed once severe anxiety has been present for at least six months) include:

- Excessive anxiety about being around other people
- Excessive feelings of self-consciousness

- Fear of being judged by others
- Worrying extensively before a social event
- Blushing, sweating or trembling when around other people
- Difficulty making and keeping friends
- Feeling nauseated when around other people
- Avoiding other people

For some people, it may become so severe that they cannot face going out alone (agoraphobia).

Obsessive-compulsive disorder (OCD) affects around one in fifty people and is no longer classed as an anxiety disorder as such, although anxiety plays a key role. It involves having persistent unwelcome thoughts (obsessions) which may force you to carry out certain rituals (compulsions) in an attempt to relieve the distress caused by the obsession. A common obsession is with germs and dirt, which leads sufferers to wash their hands repeatedly. Other examples include repeatedly checking something (such as that the oven is off), obsessively counting or arranging items or hoarding things you don't need because you fear something bad will happen if you throw them away. You are unlikely to get any pleasure from carrying out these rituals; they just provide temporary relief from the anxiety caused by the obsessive thoughts.

Many people can think of times when they have experienced an obsession, such as excessive exercise, or a compulsion, such as going back to check you locked the front door, and these are often a normal response to stress. But when they start to affect your behaviour for at least an hour of every day and cause you distress because they interfere with your daily life (for example, by making you late for work because you're checking and/or double-checking you've turned the oven off), it is very likely you are suffering from OCD.

Panic attacks can be brought on by the emotional and physical symptoms of anxiety. At first, you may only feel panicky when you are in a situation you find particularly stressful, such as flying or having to give a speech, and they may be one-off events. But sometimes they recur and become worse so that just *thinking about* what brings on the feelings of stress can trigger an overwhelming sense of panic. Sometimes panic attacks come on with no obvious underlying trigger; panic disorder is diagnosed when intense fear and other panic symptoms develop abruptly and rapidly, followed by a period of at least a month of persistent worry about the attack recurring. While many people have experienced a one-off panic attack at some time, panic disorder affects around one in fifty people.

One-off panic attacks have been linked with hyperventilation – overbreathing in which you breathe rapidly and shallowly, so you exhale more carbon dioxide (a waste gas produced by our metabolism) than normal. This changes the acid balance in our blood, interfering with the way our throat muscles move, and this can create the sensation of a lump in the throat. Overbreathing also affects the way our nerves send signals, leading to sensations of pins and needles (often felt first around the mouth), and can lead to dizziness and feeling faint. These symptoms can in themselves heighten your sense of panic, which is likely to cause you to breathe even faster, so you exhale even more carbon dioxide, which can then trigger a full-blown panic attack.

Rebreathing air you have just blown out (traditionally using a paper bag, but it's easier to use your cupped hands) helps to correct your loss of blood acidity so your symptoms improve.

Many people who only suffer occasional panic attacks learn to cope with them by using relaxation techniques and breathing exercises. If your symptoms are becoming debilitating, however, you may benefit from learning anxiety management techniques with the help of a behavioural therapist. Some antidepressant drugs can also be prescribed to help control panic disorder.

A review published in the medical journal *Current Neuropharmacology* in 2017 assessed all the research evidence, and concluded that CBD is also a promising treatment for panic disorder.[6]

How CBD can help anxiety

CBD is emerging as an effective alternative to anti-anxiety medication for mild or moderate anxiety, but there is not yet a clear consensus on exactly how effective it is. The endocannabinoid system helps to regulate the way we respond to stress by passing messages back against the usual flow of information to reduce overactive brain cells (see retrograde signalling, page 59). When this regulation goes wrong, however, anxiety can result, and anxiety disorders are increasingly thought to involve an endocannabinoid deficiency.

Studies have shown that mice that genetically lack CB1 receptors appear more anxious than normal mice, for example, which suggests that a fully working endocannabinoid system is needed to control anxiety properly – at least in rodents. People have used marijuana for hundreds, if not thousands of years, to help take the edge off anxiety and stress, which strongly suggests that the endocannabinoid system is involved in regulating anxiety in us, too.

This was highlighted in clinical trials involving rimonabant, a synthetic cannabinoid that was launched as an anti-obesity drug. Rimonabant worked by blocking the effects of CB1 receptors, but this led to an unwanted increase in anxiety and so the drug was taken off the market.[7] Rimonabant mimicked what would happen if our own endocannabinoid anandamide was no longer able to interact with CB1 receptors to suppress anxiety. Since then, studies have confirmed that people with high levels of anxiety have lower than normal levels of anandamide in their bloodstream.

CBD helps to reduce anxiety by prolonging the action of anandamide, which has an uplifting, 'blissful' effect. CBD also helps to reduce overactive thoughts and generate calm without the 'high' associated with the THC in marijuana.

What the research shows

The first suggestion that CBD reduces anxiety was published back in 1982 following a small trial involving just eight, healthy volunteers. On different occasions, the volunteers took CBD, THC, THC + CBD, a tranquilliser (diazepam) or a placebo without knowing which was which. The results showed that THC *increased* anxiety but adding in CBD significantly reduced this effect.[8]

The researchers therefore decided to investigate CBD further on its own, and to compare its effects against prescribed tranquillisers. As noted, one of the most common forms of social anxiety is a fear of public speaking. The researchers therefore designed an experiment in which volunteers (who did not have a social anxiety disorder but, like most people, preferred not to speak in public) were asked to speak in front of a video camera while their heart rate, blood pressure and other stress responses were measured. Forty people took either CBD (in quite a high dose of 300mg – only take this with your doctor's permission) or one of two anti-anxiety drugs. CBD was found to be better at reducing anxiety than one of the anti-anxiety drugs, and almost as effective as the other.[9]

CBD was then tested in a group of twenty-four people with diagnosed social anxiety who were asked to take part in a similar public-speaking test. Each person was asked to take either an even higher dose of 600mg CBD (under medical supervision) or a placebo an hour-and-a-half before the test, and their responses were compared to another group of twelve healthy volunteers who didn't take anything. Among those with social anxiety, CBD significantly reduced feelings of anxiety, muddled thoughts, negative self-judgements and discomfort during their performance compared with the placebo. They also reported that CBD helped them feel significantly calmer beforehand while they were anticipating their speech. In fact, those taking CBD performed as well as those without social anxiety when it came to changes in their blood pressure, heart rate and level of anxiety.[10]

Another study used a special type of brain scan (single-photon emission computed tomography, or SPECT) to see how CBD affected blood flow throughout the brain in ten volunteers who took either 400mg CBD or a placebo ninety minutes before the scan. CBD was found to significantly reduce feelings of anxiety during the scan and these effects were linked with changes in activity in parts of the brain that suggest it has genuine anti-anxiety effects.[11]

These results were confirmed using another type of brain scan (fMRI) in fifteen volunteers who were shown scary images in order to increase their level of anxiety. In this experiment, taking a high dose of CBD reduced activity in primitive parts of the brain that help us to respond to fear by becoming more anxious and alert.[12]

It's important to note that these effects were shown in clinical trials that used much higher doses than those recommended in this book. However, in a recent US study, doctors prescribed much lower doses of CBD to forty-seven people with anxiety instead of starting them on anti-anxiety medication or to reduce their doses (only combine CBD with medications under the advice and supervision of your own doctor). Most people in the trial took just 25mg CBD (after breakfast) while a handful received an increased dose of 50mg or 75mg CBD per day if needed. The doctors reported that CBD significantly reduced the level of anxiety in 79% of patients within the first month, and these levels remained decreased when followed up for a further two months.[13]

A 2012 review of all the clinical trial evidence involving

CBD and anxiety concluded that CBD has clear anti-anxiety effects that are similar to those of prescribed anti-anxiety drugs.[14] So, for dealing with day-to-day anxiety associated with the pressures of modern life, it is likely that CBD will help you feel more calm, relaxed and able to cope, even when taken at relatively low doses.

Do check with your doctor that CBD doesn't interact with any other medication you are taking, however.

CBD and low mood

Few of us feel happy all the time and one day we may feel cheerful, energetic and lively, and then the next day we feel gloomy for no obvious reason. These mood swings are a normal reaction to the events of everyday life, hormone swings and even seasonal changes, but if your mood swings too low, it can lead to depression.

Studies suggest that CBD can help to lift a low mood, as described below, and depression is among the top four reasons CBD users take it (alongside pain, anxiety and sleep problems).

What is depression?

Depression is a biological illness and is traditionally associated with an imbalance of brain chemicals such as serotonin, norepinephrine (also known as noradrenaline) and dopamine. Depression is a complex condition, and what triggers it and why it becomes chronic for some people while others are not affected is unknown. Factors that appear to increase the risk of depression include the genes you inherit, traumatic life events such as abuse or bereavement, developing a serious physical illness or taking certain medications such as corticosteroids. New research suggests that depletion of endocannabinoids may also play a role.

Neurotransmitters such as serotonin and dopamine pass messages from one brain cell to another across the tiny gaps (synapses) between each brain cell. Once neurotransmitters cross these gaps, they trigger an electrical response in the next brain cell to either increase or decrease its activity. These responses are what allow us to interpret the world around us, think logically and solve new problems by thinking about similar situations in the past.

After they have done their job, the neurotransmitters are then reabsorbed into the cell that released them and are broken down for recycling. If your neurotransmitter levels fall too low – because not enough are produced, or if they are cleared away too quickly – the passage of messages between brain cells does not continue as usual.

In many cases, low mood is only temporary and you bounce back within a few days. If the low mood becomes persistent, however, and lasts for at least two weeks, your doctor may diagnose you with depression. Some people experience big mood swings between depression and excessive feelings of elation, and this is known as bipolar disorder or manic depression.

Depression is common. According to the World Health Organization, it affects more than 300 million people across the globe.

The chance of experiencing a major depressive episode during your lifetime is around one in ten for men and as high as one in five for women.

It is likely that you are experiencing depression if you:

- Often feel down, depressed or hopeless
- Have little interest or pleasure in doing things, particularly things that once gave you pleasure

As well as the above two main symptoms, you may also experience:

- Fatigue or loss of energy
- Feeling generally slowed down or sluggish in your thoughts and actions
- Sleep difficulties such as waking up in the early hours
- Being unable to think straight, concentrate or make decisions
- Feeling worthless, with excessive or inappropriate feelings of guilt
- Reduced appetite and weight loss

If you are severely depressed you may have recurrent thoughts about death or have suicidal thoughts, in which case it's vital to seek medical help urgently.

Helplines

If you think you may be depressed, it is important to tell your doctor. You can also contact the following helplines who provide emotional support to help prevent suicide:

UK: Samaritans, samaritans.org. Tel: 116 123 around the clock, twenty-four hours a day, 365 days a year.

Befrienders Worldwide: find your country's helpline at www.befrienders.org.

If you think you are depressed, visit your doctor and tell him or her how you're feeling. They will assess your symptoms and decide which of the following treatments you will benefit from:

- Ongoing monitoring with regular assessment and support from your GP. If your symptoms are mild your doctor will provide advice and arrange follow-up within one to two weeks to see if you are getting better or worse
- Psychological therapies such as individual guided self-help, group-based therapies, physical activity programmes or cognitive behavioural therapy (CBT)
- Antidepressant drugs such as SSRIs (selective serotonin reuptake inhibitors) are no longer used routinely for mild depression. They may be offered alongside psychological therapy if you are experiencing moderate to severe depression

If your doctor has not prescribed antidepressant drugs, he or she may agree to support you while you try a CBD oil supplement (drops, spray or capsules) as a self-help treatment, under their supervision, with regular reviews to ensure you are improving rather than getting worse.

The endocannabinoid system and depression

Laboratory studies have shown that stimulation of CB1 cannabinoid receptors in the brain has an antidepressant effect and this is one of the ways in which our endocannabinoid anandamide helps to lift our mood. Anandamide also has beneficial effects on the mood-lifting action of other brain chemicals (neurotransmitters) such as serotonin and dopamine.

When our mood starts to swing low, our endocannabinoids help to stimulate some underactive pathways, and when our mood swings too high they help to damp down other overactive pathways to keep our emotions on a more even keel. If this damping-down action of the endocannabinoid system becomes too dominant, however, it's possible that it might lead to depression.

People with depression who use medical marijuana (containing THC plus CBD) often claim that it helps to stabilise their mood, lift their depression and, in those with bipolar disorder, that it also relieves episodes of mania (the overactive euphoric phase of bipolar or manic depression). Psychiatrists noted this back in 2005 and called for studies to investigate these effects, but so far no clinical trials have been published. At the time of writing, at least thirty-six clinical trials into CBD, medical marijuana and mental health conditions are underway globally that may help to shed more light on the situation.

What the research shows

CBD is emerging as a natural antidepressant with potential benefits in clinical depression and anhedonia – the inability to feel pleasure in normally pleasurable activities. As well as interacting with cannabinoid receptors and prolonging the effects of our anandamide, CBD also interacts with serotonin receptors to help lift a low mood. Serotonin is often referred to as our 'happy chemical' as it helps us to feel upbeat and well.

One of the ways in which researchers measure the effects of an antidepressant drug is to measure levels of a substance known as BDNF (brain-derived neurotrophic factor), which fall in people who are depressed and rise again when they take antidepressant medications. The way that CBD affects BDNF levels was assessed in a laboratory study published in 2019. This showed that administering CBD caused a rapid rise in BDNF levels within thirty minutes and also had an antidepressant effect – suggesting that CBD has a rapid and sustained antidepressant action. In fact, its effects were so rapid that a single dose produced a measurable response, while prescribed antidepressant drugs (SSRIs) typically take two or more weeks to produce a noticeable effect.[15]

As these results involve rodents they need to be approached with some caution. This research is so recent that gold-standard clinical trials have not yet assessed the effects of CBD on mild to moderate depression in human volunteers. Even so, the research that is available, as well as anecdotal reports, suggest that CBD can help to lift a low mood. If you want to try CBD for depression, do speak to your doctor first so they can monitor whether or not your symptoms are improving.

CBD and sleep

Insomnia and sleep disorders are among the top four reasons for taking CBD. Even if you don't consider yourself to have a sleep problem, you may notice – like myself – that you sleep more deeply and wake feeling more refreshed when taking CBD at night.

Sleep is a natural form of unconsciousness in which parts of the brain switch off but other areas become more active. During sleep, our brain processes information and experiences to lay down new memories. Our muscles and joints recover from constant use during the day and we produce increased amounts of growth hormone, which stimulates the regeneration and rejuvenation of our cells. As a result, protein in all parts of the body is replenished faster, and you produce new cells more quickly when you are asleep than when you are awake. Sleep is also the time when our immune cells return from the bloodstream to our lymph nodes where they are reprogrammed and activated to fight infection.

Getting just the right amount of sleep is therefore important for long-term good health and immunity. Sleep disorders are common, however, and of the seven different types that are recognised, insomnia – the inability to fall asleep or stay asleep – is by far the most common.

Some sleep disorders are now thought to result from an endocannabinoid deficiency – especially those affecting rapid eye movement (REM) sleep, which is the stage of sleep in which you dream.

The different stages of sleep

We experience two main phases of sleep: rapid eye movement (REM) sleep, in which our eyes are constantly on the move, and slow-wave (or non-REM) sleep, in which our eyes are relatively still. Slow-wave sleep is itself divided into two stages, one of light sleep and one of deep sleep. The most restorative stages of sleep are deep sleep and REM sleep rather than light sleep.

When we first fall asleep, we pass through the lightest stage of sleep to reach the deeper stages. Sleep then lightens again and we spend a period of around ten minutes in REM sleep, although it can occur at any time during sleep. This cycle typically lasts ninety to 120 minutes and we typically go through four or five of these sleep cycles throughout the night.

For most of us, light sleep makes up 40 to 60% of our total sleep time, while deep sleep makes up 5 to 15% of our total sleep time. REM sleep typically begins ninety minutes after you first fall asleep and, as morning approaches, we spend more and more time – up to one hour – in REM sleep (which is important for laying down memories). The rest of the time we spend in slow-wave sleep.

Interestingly, people who only sleep four hours per night get a similar amount of slow-wave sleep as those who regularly sleep eight hours per night – additional time asleep is spent in REM sleep, in which the brain refreshes and restores itself so you feel more mentally recharged. If someone is woken during REM sleep, they will usually say they've been dreaming. This is also the phase of sleep in which some people grind their teeth.

Sleep Efficiency

We sometimes hear about 'sleep efficiency' when we talk about difficulty sleeping. Sleep efficiency is measured as the total time we spend asleep divided by the total time we spend in bed. If you fall asleep as soon as you get into bed and have a good night's sleep, you will have a high sleep efficiency of at least 90%. But if you toss and turn before nodding off, then wake several times during the night, your sleep efficiency will be low (considered to be less than 70%).

Sleep problems

Insomnia is a difficulty in falling asleep, or staying asleep, and when you do manage to nod off, the quality of your sleep is not restorative so your ability to function during the following day is affected. Most of us have suffered from insomnia at some stage of our lives – usually when we are worried about something or stressed.

Lying awake in bed, despite feeling tired and in desperate need of sleep, is a miserable experience. As well as affecting our emotional wellbeing, poor quality sleep increases the risk of having an accident (due to excessive tiredness), raises our blood pressure, and reduces our immunity so we are less able to fight off infections. If you are exposed to a common cold virus, for example, you are almost three times more likely to catch it and develop symptoms if you consistently get less than seven hours of sleep a night, than if you were sleeping eight hours or more. Getting too little REM sleep can also lead to difficulty concentrating, poor memory, irritability and anxiety.

The endocannabinoid system (ECS) is closely linked to our sleep–wake cycle and body clock – the natural circadian rhythms or cyclic changes that occur over a twenty-four-hour period in response to light and dark. Examples of body functions that show a circadian rhythm and which change according to the time of day or night include sleep, body temperature and hormone levels.

When levels of the endocannabinoid anandamide were measured in the blood of five healthy volunteers they were shown to be three times higher on waking than immediately before going to sleep, indicating a strong connection to the natural circadian rhythm. Following a night in which the volunteers weren't allowed to sleep, however, this natural rhythm did not occur and there were no differences in their blood levels of anandamide between evening and morning. This suggests that lack of normal sleep can profoundly affect the natural way that anandamide levels change to reflect the time of day. Laboratory studies also show that the number of CB1 receptors significantly increases in parts of the brain when we are sleep-deprived and this may be a protective response to help us recover from the harmful effects of lack of sleep.

What does the research show?

Preliminary studies are starting to show that taking CBD can help to normalise sleep patterns, restore REM sleep and reduce excessive daytime sleepiness.[17] CBD also helps you get a good night's sleep when you are stressed by reducing muscle tension, restlessness and anxiety.

Research dating back to the 1970s investigated the effects of marijuana on sleep and produced mixed findings. Some studies found marijuana helped people fall asleep, some showed it increased waking after falling asleep, while others found it affected the sleep cycle by increasing slow-wave sleep and decreasing REM sleep. However, other studies found no effects at all.

These conflicting results appeared to relate to the THC – you start to become immune to its effects when using it regularly so that it becomes less effective and the short-term benefits on sleep are lost. As a result, users could find themselves in a vicious cycle of having to use more and more cannabis to manage their sleep. This increased use could also lead to withdrawal symptoms, which can in turn cause sleep disturbances and vivid dreams, making the situation worse.[18]

If THC is removed from the equation, however, the effects of CBD can shine. CBD helps to regulate your sleep–wake cycle so that you fall asleep more easily, without causing a hangover effect the next day (as many prescribed sleeping tablets do). Early studies from the 1980s used relatively high doses of 160mg CBD which were found to increase sleep quality so that people fell asleep more quickly, stayed asleep for longer and slept more soundly through the night, whether they were healthy volunteers, insomniacs or people with epilepsy. You don't need such a high dose, however, as research also shows that lower doses of 40mg and 80mg CBD also improved deep sleep and REM sleep with less dream recall, which suggests that the last phase of refreshing REM sleep was completed before waking.[19]

In other studies, CBD improved sleep in two thirds of people who took 25mg of CBD after dinner.[20] Even lower doses can help. A recent study presented at the sixteenth annual conference of the International Society of Sports Nutrition in 2019 showed that taking just 15mg CBD for six weeks produced significant improvements in sleep and quality of life, such as less daytime sleepiness.[21]

Using CBD to aid sleep

I find that taking just one 6.4mg CBD capsule at night on getting into bed works really well for me. I start reading and within twenty minutes my eyelids begin to droop. This dose is enough to promote a deep and refreshing night's sleep and I don't recall my dreams. This suggests that I complete my last REM cycle and don't wake during my last REM sleep (which is when you dream). When I increased the dose to 15mg CBD, however, I had some very vivid dreams (suggesting I was not completing my last sleep cycle and was waking during REM sleep) so I dropped back to the 6.4mg dose.

Some wrist activity monitors can detect the different stages of sleep based on the degree of movement they sense and variations in your heart rate. This can give an accurate picture of how taking CBD affects the quality of your sleep.

If you want to see how CBD affects the quality of your sleep, read the chapter on taking CBD safely to ensure you select a good quality product, then start with a low dose of CBD, half an hour before bedtime. After a few nights, you can increase the dose if necessary until you find what works best for you.

Tips to help you wake up feeling better:

- Avoid napping during the day as this will make it more difficult to sleep at night
- Take regular exercise during the day but avoid strenuous exercise in the evening which will keep you awake
- Eat your evening meal before 7pm and resist late-night snacks, especially of rich food
- Eat a protein-rich diet and avoid getting hungry, as this will keep you alert and make it difficult to fall asleep
- Avoid substances known to interfere with sleep such as caffeine (coffee, tea, chocolate, colas), nicotine and alcohol – although alcohol may help you fall asleep initially, you are likely to have a disturbed sleep once the anaesthetic-like effect wears off
- Take time to unwind from the stresses of the day before going to bed – read a book, listen to soothing music or have a candlelit bath

- A warm, milky drink just before going to bed will help you to relax – hot milk with cinnamon or nutmeg is better than chocolatey drinks that contain some caffeine
- Don't drink too much fluid in the evening – a full bladder is guaranteed to disturb your rest
- Get into a habit by going to bed at a regular time each night and getting up at the same time each morning
- Set a bedtime routine such as locking up, brushing your teeth, bathing and setting the alarm clock to get yourself in the mood for sleep
- Make sure your bed is comfortable and your bedroom warm, dark and quiet – noise and excessive cold or heat will keep you awake. A temperature of 18–24°C is ideal
- Keep your bedroom as a place for sleep – don't use it for eating, working or watching television
- Make sure all your electrical devices are at least 6 feet away from your bed as they may emit electromagnetic frequencies that interfere with sleep. Unplug devices when not in use
- Don't use an electronic screen before sleep. The blue light emitted by smartphones, tablets and similar devices switch off the production of melatonin – your natural sleep hormone. Read an old-fashioned book before sleep rather than using an e-reader
- If you can't sleep, don't lie there tossing and turning. Get up and read for a while. If you are worried about something, write down all the things on your mind and promise yourself you will deal with them in the morning, when you are feeling fresher. When you feel sleepy,

go back to bed and try again. If sleep does not come within fifteen minutes, get up and repeat this process

CBD and quitting smoking

The legendary Sir Francis Drake has a lot to answer for. After circumnavigating the globe, he returned from the Americas in 1573 with the first consignment of tobacco to hit English shores. Smoking quickly became a fashionable necessity for socialites and it was almost 400 years before the habit was recognised as harmful – not just for those actively smoking, but for those passively inhaling the smoke, too.

More than 1 billion of us smoke cigarettes worldwide and an estimated 8 million people die every year as a direct result. According to the World Health Organization, tobacco will eventually kill up to half of its users, making it the single greatest cause of preventable death across the globe. In fact, the reduction in mortality due to not smoking is so great that being a non-smoker can add an estimated fourteen years to your life span.

Cigarettes are harmful because the burning of tobacco leaves exposes you to over 4,000 different chemicals of which at least sixty are carcinogenic and 400 are toxic. Unfortunately, quitting is difficult because the nicotine found in tobacco – which produces pleasant feelings – is highly addictive. Surveys suggest that four out of five smokers want to give up, and have tried many times, but the nicotine withdrawal symptoms of tension, aggression, depression and insomnia, plus the cravings, make it difficult to stop even though you know it's harming you. People who follow a quit plan (a series of steps designed to help them stop smoking) and who slowly reduce their intake of nicotine using nicotine replacement products (such as patches, chewing gum, sprays, microtabs or inhaled forms) are at least twice as likely to succeed as those who just stop abruptly and 'go cold turkey' – a phrase derived from the goose pimples that can develop when you kick a habit. This is where CBD may help.

In studies, CBD helps to reduce the food cravings caused by THC.[22] As these cravings are similar in nature to those felt by people quitting nicotine, researchers wanted to see if CBD could also help to block nicotine cravings. In one study, twenty-four people who smoked at least ten cigarettes a day, and who wanted to quit, were given an inhaler which delivered either CBD or a placebo. They were asked to use their inhaler whenever they felt like smoking and to record their daily cigarette and inhaler use in a diary for one week. The results showed a 'dramatic' reduction of 40% in the number of cigarettes smoked in those using the CBD inhaler, without any increase in cigarette cravings. In contrast, those using a placebo inhaler showed no difference in the number of cigarettes smoked compared with their normal intake.[23]

The researchers concluded that these were very encouraging findings, given how cravings usually lead to smokers relapsing when trying to quit cigarettes. However, they cautioned that larger studies with longer follow-up are needed to confirm that CBD can help smokers to quit.

If you want to quit smoking cigarettes, then CBD may help you succeed. I recommend using CBD as an oral spray (starting with one spray and, if needed, increasing until you reach the manufacturer's maximum recommended dose), or a few drops held under the tongue. Use the CBD spray or drops whenever you feel like smoking and keep a record of the number of CBD uses and the number of cigarettes you smoke. This diary will help to focus your mind and maintain your motivation. While you can use a CBD vape instead, do read about the dangers of vaping on page 117 first before deciding whether or not this is the best option for you.

You can use an oral CBD supplement to help wean you off nicotine replacement therapy, too. You can use CBD together with a nicotine patch to combat withdrawal symptoms.

As a doctor, I am convinced of the many benefits of CBD supplements on the many physical and emotional conditions covered in this book. Everyone is different, however, and not all of us will respond in the same way when taking CBD. If CBD is not producing the improvements you are looking for, or if you are not able to take CBD because of the prescribed medicines you are taking, then PEA is a useful alternative to help reduce pain, stiffness and inflammation, as we will examine in chapter nine.

8

Hemp Seed Oil

Hemp seed oil is often added to CBD supplements to produce a CBD oil that is wholly derived from the non-drug strains of cannabis, known as industrial hemp. While CBD is found in the green parts of hemp plants, hemp seed oil is pressed from the seeds. Pure hemp seed oil should not contain any cannabinoids such as CBD or THC, but these are often present in significant amounts (see page 250), which is why hemp seed oil is included here.

The nutritional value of hemp seed oil

Hemp seed oil is a healthy, nutritionally balanced oil that provides a high level of 'good' monounsaturated fats (similar to those found in olive oil), plus essential fatty acids with only a low level of saturated fat. It is considered nutritionally balanced as it provides a three-to-one ratio of the two essential types of fatty acids – omega-6s and omega-3s. Just one tablespoon (15ml) of hemp seed oil provides your daily requirement of essential fatty acids. Hemp seed oil is also rich in plant sterols (which lower cholesterol) and vitamin E.

Essential Fatty Acids

Essential fatty acids are so called because they can't be made in the body and must therefore come from your diet. They are mainly found in nuts, seeds and their oils, and in seafood. You need essential fatty acids to make cell membranes, sex hormones and hormone-like chemicals (prostaglandins) that help to control inflammatory reactions.

When essential fatty acids are in short supply, you are more likely to develop dry, itchy skin, flare-ups of chronic inflammatory diseases (e.g. rheumatoid arthritis, psoriasis, eczema or asthma), and women are more likely to have painful periods. As these are all conditions for which CBD is also helpful, a CBD oil that includes hemp seed oil provides additional benefits.

Hemp seed oil has a deep green colour and a nutty, buttery flavour that has been described as similar to a blend of pine nut and sesame seed oil. Different hemp seed oils have different flavours, however, and some can taste quite grassy or earthy.

As hemp seed oil has a low smoke point, it isn't used for cooking or frying, but to drizzle over food and to add to salad dressings, dips and pesto sauce. It is also used to make soaps, skin lotions, shampoo and biofuels.

One acre of hemp plants can yield between 800 and 1,000 pounds of seed.

Cannabinoids in hemp seed oil

The amount of plant cannabinoids (phytocannabinoids) found in plain hemp seed oil should be very low, as the kernels contain only trace amounts of THC and CBD. However, the outside of the seed coat becomes contaminated by rubbing against the resinous glands of the upper leaves during maturation, harvesting, and processing. This can lead to detectable levels of CBD and THC in hemp seed oil products, although this will not usually be indicated on the label unless the oil is tested (which most aren't).

When eight hemp seed oils were tested in the US (some bottled oils, some capsules) all had detectable levels of THC, some at high concentrations. Consuming large amounts of these hemp seed oils (more than one tablespoon) could produce a positive result in drug tests that detect THC in urine.[1]

Some hemp seed oils tested in Croatia had such high levels of THC that they were almost certainly made from illegal marijuana strains of cannabis rather than from industrial hemp.[2]

So, if you are subject to random urine drug tests, and/or want to avoid THC, you may prefer not to use hemp seed oil, or to only buy hemp oils that have been tested and labelled as having undetectable amounts of THC (below three parts per million). Otherwise, if this is not an issue for you, you may find that the small amounts of cannabinoids found in hemp seed oil add to its therapeutic benefits.

Medicinal benefits of hemp seed oil

Hemp seed oil is traditionally used to correct hormone imbalances and to improve skin conditions but it is now increasingly used in general skincare moisturisers, too. People who have taken hemp seed oil supplements for several months have reported that their skin becomes softer and less dry, their fingernails grow stronger and their hair becomes thicker and more glossy.

Hemp seed oil has been used for centuries in Chinese and Korean medicine to treat inflammatory conditions such as eczema and rheumatoid arthritis.

In Finland, hemp seed oil is often used to treat eczema (atopic dermatitis) but this use is based on anecdote and word of mouth rather than medical evidence. Finnish dermatologists therefore compared the effects of hemp seed oil against olive oil in twenty patients with eczema, who took two tablespoons (30ml) of either hemp seed oil or olive oil every day for eight weeks. After a break, they then took the other oil for another eight weeks to compare the effects of the two. When taking the hemp seed oil, their eczema significantly improved, with reduced itching and dryness so they needed to use less emollient (softening and moisturising) creams compared with the time during which they took the olive oil.[3] This has led to some doctors recommending it as, despite the low level of clinical evidence, it is a nutritionally valuable oil and there is no harm in trying it to see if it helps a skin problem.

The anti-inflammatory effects of hemp seed oil may also offer some benefits to people with multiple sclerosis, according to promising findings from one clinical trial. When 100 people with multiple sclerosis took hemp seed oil for six months, their symptoms improved and they were less likely to have a relapse of symptoms than when they took olive oil.[4] CBD and medical marijuana also have beneficial effects in people with multiple sclerosis.

If you have raised cholesterol, then taking two tablespoons (30ml) of hemp seed oil per day may help to improve your cholesterol balance by raising levels of 'good' HDL-cholesterol and lowering levels of other forms of 'bad' cholesterol. This effect is due to the plant sterols that are naturally found in hemp seed oil and which block the absorption of cholesterol in the gut. As a result, less cholesterol reaches the liver for processing and less of the 'bad' forms of cholesterol are released back into the bloodstream.

So, when choosing a CBD oil supplement, those that include hemp seed oil are a good choice if you have a raised cholesterol or an inflammatory skin condition such as eczema. You can also use hemp seed oil in the kitchen for making salad dressings or drizzling over food to help provide the essential fatty acids you need for good health.

9

PEA – the New CBD Alternative

Some people are unable to take CBD because it interferes with the effects of prescribed medicines they are taking or they have to undergo drug testing and don't want to risk having detectable levels of THC in their blood or urine. Some people also feel uncomfortable taking CBD because it comes from cannabis plants. It's therefore good to know that an alternative supplement provides similar benefits to CBD and is not known to interact with any prescribed medications. Also, because it does not come from hemp plants, there is no chance of the supplement containing any trace levels of THC that might affect urine drugs testing.

This supplement is known as PEA, which is short for palmitoylethanolamide. PEA is found naturally in some foods such as milk, soybeans, alfalfa, peanuts and egg yolks, but the PEA used in supplements is made from palmitic acid from sustainably sourced palm trees.

The PEA found in supplements is identical to the PEA we make ourselves. While PEA is not classed as an endocannabinoid because it does not act directly on our endocannabinoid receptors (CB1 and CB2), it can be considered as a component of the endocannabinoid system as it enhances the effects of our main endocannabinoid, anandamide. PEA is naturally made in our bodies by cells as part of our biological response to pain and inflammation. It is produced whenever we cut ourselves or experience a sports injury, burn, frostbite, infection or allergic reaction, for example, and is also produced as part of the healing response in chronic inflammatory conditions such as rheumatoid arthritis.

PEA supplements have been widely researched and, like CBD, can help to reduce pain and inflammation and aid relaxation and sleep.[1] This makes PEA particularly popular among athletes who don't want to use CBD products in case they inadvertently consume even a small amount of THC, which is a banned drug in elite sports.

PEA and pain

PEA has a powerful analgesic effect against many different types of chronic and neurological pain, including neuralgia, diabetic neuropathy, sciatica, carpel tunnel syndrome and other trapped nerve conditions. Eight clinical studies, involving over a thousand people, have confirmed that taking PEA produces significantly greater pain relief in a wide range of conditions than placebo.[2]

Another analysis of twelve studies found that taking PEA produces a progressive reduction in pain so that, on average, discomfort was reduced by one point (on a zero to ten pain intensity score, see page 142) every two weeks. Eight out of ten people taking PEA supplements reported a significant reduction in pain within two months of treatment.[3]

PEA is particularly helpful for painful osteoarthritis of the knee. For example, in an Australian study, 111 volunteers took either 300mg PEA or 600mg PEA daily (divided into two doses, or a placebo, for eight weeks. In those taking PEA, their level of pain and stiffness significantly improved compared with those taking placebo. Interestingly, they also reported feeling less anxious.[4]

PEA and sleep

By interacting with our natural endocannabinoids, PEA helps to regulate our sleep–wake cycle (circadian rhythms) and, in some animals, is involved in hibernation. PEA has a calming and relaxing effect and promotes restful and restorative REM (rapid eye movement) sleep (see page 238). It also improves sleep by reducing inflammation and pain which can keep us awake. In people with carpal tunnel syndrome, for example, sleep is often fragmented, but taking PEA supplements reduced pain intensity and helped sufferers fall asleep more quickly, spend more time continuously asleep and wake up feeling more refreshed.

PEA and stress

During times of physical or emotional stress, the production of anandamide and PEA increases. This helps to reduce anxiety and also helps us to forget particularly traumatic events. People with high blood levels of PEA appear to have a higher tolerance to stress and are less likely to become depressed or to experience post-traumatic stress than those with lower PEA levels.[6] This suggests that taking PEA supplements may improve our resilience to stress, although this has not yet been tested in clinical trials.

PEA and eczema

Like our endocannabinoids, PEA is made in skin cells and it is already used in veterinary medicine to treat a variety of inflammatory and scaly skin conditions. When tested in sixty people with eczema, adding PEA to emollient (moisturising) skin creams for twenty-eight days improved itching, dryness, roughness and scaling, as well as boosting skin hydration.[7]

Evidence for the effectiveness of PEA is building, with studies starting to assess its effects in other chronic inflammatory diseases such as asthma, in neuropathic pain and in some neurological conditions such as multiple sclerosis, Alzheimer's and Parkinson's disease.[8] Large clinical trials are needed to confirm its role in these conditions, but it appears to be a safe supplement. When used in doses of 200mg to 600mg per day, no serious side effects or drug interactions have so far been reported.

As a result of all these studies PEA is gaining in popularity, particularly among people who prefer not to take a cannabis-based product such as CBD. Athletes, for example, who are subjected to drugs testing and don't want to risk taking a supplement that may contain traces of the banned phytocannabinoid, THC, are increasingly turning to PEA for relaxation and to help reduce muscle and joint aches and pains resulting from intense training. If CBD is withdrawn at any time as a result of the uncertainty over the EU novel foods regulations, then PEA is nicely positioned to act as a replacement.

*

I hope you have found the information about PEA, CBD and medical marijuana in this book helpful. New research is being published daily and our understanding of the health and wellness benefits of CBD in particular is rapidly expanding. If you haven't yet taken a CBD supplement then I hope the studies covered in this book will help to guide your decision on whether or not to try it. As always, if you have a medical condition or are taking prescribed drugs, do check with your doctor first and follow their advice.

Acknowledgements

Thanks, as always, to my family for providing vital support throughout the long hours I spent holed up in my study reading the many research publications relating to CBD. Thanks also to my agents, Watson Little, and to my editor, Fritha Saunders, whose unfailing enthusiasm and constructive suggestions have helped to make this book so much better.

Glossary

2-AG (2-arachidonoylglycerol) – one of the main two endo-cannabinoids made in our body.

Anandamide (N-arachidonoylethanolamide) – one of the main two endocannabinoids made in our body. It is named after the Sanskrit word *ananda*, meaning 'bliss' or 'supreme joy' due to its uplifting effects on our mood.

Antioxidant – a protective substance that helps to neutralise damaging chemical reactions (known as oxidation) in the body.

Atherosclerosis – hardening and furring up of the arteries, which causes them to narrow due to a build-up of cholesterol-laden deposits known as plaques.

Cannabidiol (CBD) – a plant cannabinoid that is the most common cannabinoid in hemp strains of cannabis plants. In marijuana strains of the cannabis plant, CBD is among the top two most common cannabinoids. Most marijuana strains contain more tetrahydrocannabinol (THC) than CBD, but some contain similar amounts and a few contain more CBD than THC. CBD is non-intoxicating and does not cause a 'high'.

Cannabidiolic acid (CBDA) – an inactive molecule found in cannabis plants which converts into cannabidiol (CBD) in a process known as decarboxylation.

Cannabinoids – a group of chemicals that were originally discovered in cannabis plants. These include THC and CBD.

Cannabinol (CBN) – a mildly psychoactive cannabinoid that forms from the breakdown of THC. It is usually only present in trace amounts but levels can rise in aged cannabis plants.

Cannabis – can refer to cannabis plants (whose botanical name is *Cannabis sativa* L.), or to the psychoactive (mind-altering) herbal preparations derived from cannabis plants that are used as recreational or medicinal drugs. See *marijuana*.

CBD – see *cannabidiol*.

CBD oil – made by combining CBD with an oil (such as hemp seed oil, coconut oil or olive oil) to make increasingly popular wellness products.

Central nervous system – the part of the nervous system that co-ordinates the movement and function of the body. It is made up of the brain and spinal cord.

Clinical studies – those that involve human volunteers, whether healthy people or those who have a particular medical condition.

Decarboxylation – a chemical reaction in which unstable acidic molecules (such as CBDA) release carbon dioxide to form more stable molecules (such as CBD). This reaction is hastened by exposure to air, light or heat.

Endocannabinoid system – a communication network in our body that consists of our natural endocannabinoids, their receptors and the enzymes needed to make and recycle them.

Endocannabinoids – cannabinoids that are made naturally in our body (*endo* comes from the Greek word *endon*, meaning 'internal'). These include anandamide and 2-AG.

Extract – a plant component that is removed (or extracted) to produce a supplement.

Free radical – an unstable molecular fragment that carries a negative electrical charge in the form of a spare electron. Free radicals trigger potentially harmful chemical reactions known as oxidation.

Hashish – a cannabis resin traditionally made by collecting the sticky, hair-like glands (trichomes) and 'crystals' found on the outside of cannabis plants.

Hemp or **industrial hemp** – strains of cannabis plant that do not produce intoxicating effects as they have only low levels of THC.

Hemp oil, hemp extract oil, active hemp oil – along with similar terms are used to describe CBD oil products in jurisdictions where the legality of CBD is uncertain.

Hemp seed oil – a non-intoxicating and nutritious oil obtained from hemp strains of cannabis plants.

Homeostasis – the process (or system of checks and balances) that keeps the internal environment of the body as constant as possible. Homeostasis maintains a stable temperature, salt and fluid balance, and helps to keep the level of oxygen, glucose and other substances found in the bloodstream within safe, normal ranges.

Hormone – a chemical messenger that, when released into

the bloodstream by cells in one part of the body, has an effect on cells in another part of the body.

Marijuana – the popular term for a mind-altering drug made by drying the resinous flower buds and leaves of female cannabis plants. Marijuana is usually smoked, vaped, made into a tea or added to baked goods. The intoxicating effects of marijuana are due to THC.

Medical cannabis – any cannabis-based extract used to help relieve medical conditions such as anxiety or pain. This term can include products that are intoxicating (marijuana) or non-intoxicating (CBD) as both are derived from cannabis plants. In practice, however, the term medical cannabis usually refers to medical marijuana.

Medical marijuana – the use of the intoxicating herbal drug, marijuana, to help relieve symptoms caused by medical conditions.

Metabolism – the sum of all the chemical and physical reactions that enable the body to live, grow and function.

Neuron – a specialised cell within the nervous system that can generate and transmit electrical impulses.

Neuropathic pain – pain caused by damage to a nerve.

Neurotransmitter – a chemical that is released by a nerve or brain cell to pass signals to neighbouring cells across a communication gap known as a synapse.

Oxidation – a chemical reaction in the body that involves free radicals – unstable molecular fragments that carry a negative electric charge. This charge is passed on to other molecules which are then said to be oxidised. Oxidation reactions are linked with premature ageing and disease.

Peripheral nervous system – the part of the nervous system that connects the central nervous system (the brain and spinal cord) to the limbs and organs of the body.

Phytocannabinoids – cannabinoids that are obtained from cannabis plants (*phyto* comes from the Greek word *phyton*, meaning 'plant-grown').

Preclinical studies – studies that involve cells grown in a laboratory or animals such as mice and rats.

Receptors – special structures found on and inside our cells that detect a particular signal (such as a hormone). When activated they produce a change in that cell.

Recreational marijuana – the use of marijuana (cannabis) for relaxation or purely to obtain a mind-altering 'high' or 'stoned' effect, rather than to help relieve medical symptoms.

Synapse – the gap connection between two nerve cells. Communication across this gap may occur with the release of chemicals (neurotransmitters) or, in some cases, by an electrical message jumping across.

Tetrahydrocannabinol (THC) – a plant cannabinoid that accounts for the 'high' associated with marijuana. THC is found in marijuana (drug) strains of cannabis plants, while hemp strains have only trace levels of THC.

Tetrahydrocannabinolic acid (THCA) – an inactive molecule found in cannabis plants which converts into tetrahydrocannabinol (THC) in a process known as decarboxylation.

THC – see *tetrahydrocannabinol*.

Trichomes – hair-like glands on mature cannabis plants that produce a sticky resin that is rich in phytocannabinoids.

Further Resources

CBD and drug interactions:
CBD has the potential to interact with many prescribed and herbal medicines. Always check for interactions via your doctor or pharmacist. If they are unable to help, there is a useful drug interactions checker at Drugs.com which includes cannabidiol.

More information on accessing medical cannabis in the UK is available from:
- The United Patients Alliance: www.upalliance.org
- The Cannabis Patient Advocacy & Support Service: www.cannpass.org.
- www.drsarahbrewer.com
- The national medical cannabis registry: www.drugscience.org.uk/projecttwenty21

More information on accessing medical cannabis elsewhere in the world is available from:
marijuanadoctors.com/medical-marijuana
marijuanadoctors.com/international-patients

If you are experiencing suicidal thoughts:

Contact your doctor immediately if you have thoughts about suicide or dying. You can also find help via:

UK: Samaritans, samaritans.org. Tel: 116 123 around the clock, twenty-four hours a day, 365 days a year.

Befrienders Worldwide: find your country's helpline at www.befrienders.org.

References

1. An Introduction to Cannabidiol

1 World Health Organization, 'Cannabidiol (CBD) Pre-Review Report' (2017)
2 World Health Organization, 'Cannabidiol (CBD) Critical Review Report', Expert Committee on Drug Dependence, fortieth meeting, Geneva, 4–7 June 2018
3 Fior Markets, 'Global Industrial Hemp Market is Expected to Reach USD 14.67 Billion By 2026', 8 July 2019
4 Gibbs B et al, 'CBD in the UK: Towards a responsible, innovative and high-quality cannabidiol industry. Executive Summary', Centre for Medicinal Cannabis, 27 June 2019
5 Tim K et al, 'The Therapeutic Potential of the Phytocannabinoid Cannabidiol for Alzheimer's Disease', *Behavioural Pharmacology*, 28, 2 and 3-Spec Issue (2017):142–160
6 Corroon J, Phillips J A, 'A Cross-Sectional Study of Cannabidiol Users', *Cannabis and Cannabinoid Research*, 3 1 (2018):152–161
7 Gill L L, 'CBD Goes Mainstream', consumerreports.org, 11 April 2019

2. CBD and Medical Marijuana

1 Miller R J, Miller R E, 'Is cannabis an Effective Treatment for Joint Pain?', *Clinical and Experimental Rheumatology*, 35,

Suppl 107, 5 (2017):59–67; and European Industrial Hemp Association, 'Status of Hemp Extracts in Europe', *EIHA Press Notes*, Brussels, May 2019

2 Aizpurua-Olaizola O et al, 'Evolution of the Cannabinoid and Terpene Content During the Growth of *cannabis sativa* Plants from Different Chemotypes', *Journal of Natural Products*, 79, 2 (2016):324–31

3 Gaoni Y, Mechoulam R, 'Isolation, Structure, and Partial Synthesis of an Active Constituent of Hashish', *Journal of the American Chemical Society*, 86, 8 (1964):1646–1647

4 Grand View Research, 'Medical Marijuana Market Size to Reach USD 55.8 Billion By 2025', January 2017

5 Department of Health and Social Care, 'Cannabis: Prescriptions: Written Question – 284234', parliament.uk, 9 September 2019

6 Ware M A et al, 'The Medicinal Use of Cannabis in the UK: Results of a Nationwide Survey', *International Journal of Clinical Practice*, 59, 3 (2005):291–5

7 Centre for Medicinal Cannabis, 'NICE Guidelines Response', thecmcuk.org, 10 November 2019

8 Drug Science, 'Medicinal Cannabis: Project Twenty21', drugscience.org.uk, 7 November 2019

9 The United States Department of Justice, 'Justice Department Announces Update to Marijuana Enforcement Policy', justice.gov, 29 August 2013

10 National Conference of State Legislatures, 'State Medical Marijuana Laws', NCSL.org, 16 October 2019

11 'Number of Legal Medical Marijuana Patients', ProCon.org, 17 May 2018

12 DiForti M et al, 'The Contribution of Cannabis Use to Variation in the Incidence of Psychotic Disorder across Europe (EU-GEI): A multicentre case-control study', *Lancet Psychiatry*, 6, 5 (2019):427–436

13 American Heart Association Press Release, 'Cannabis may be linked to strokes and heart rhythm disturbances in young people', 11 November 2019.

14 'The U.S. Hemp Industry grows to $820m in sales in 2017', *Hemp Business Journal*, 2018

15 'Natural and Specialty Retail Hemp-Derived CBD Sales Projected to Grow by More Than 600% by 2022', *Hemp Business Journal*, 2018

16 Devinsky O et al, 'Efficacy and Safety of Epidiolex (Cannabidiol) in Children and Young Adults with

References

Treatment-resistant Epilepsy: Initial data from an expanded access program', *American Epilepsy Society Annual Meeting Asbtracts*, Abstract 3.303 (2014)

17 'Zimulti approval status', drugs.com, accessed 30 November 2019

3. CBD and the Endocannabinoid System

1 Di Marzo V et al, 'Endocannabinoids: Endogenous cannabinoid receptor ligands with neuromodulatory action', *Trends in Neurosciences*, 21, 12 (1998):521–8

2 Mechoulam R et al, 'Identification of an Endogenous 2-monoglyceride, Present in Canine Gut, that Binds to Cannabinoid Receptors', *Biochemcial Pharmacology*, 50, 1 (1995):83–90

3 Alger B E, 'Retrograde Signaling in the Regulation of Synaptic Transmission: Focus on Endocannabinoids', *Progress in Neurobiology*, 68, 4 (2002):247–86; and Kreitzer A C, Regehr W G, 'Retrograde Signaling by Endocannabinoids', *Current Opinion in Neurobiology*, 12, 3 (2002):324–30

4 Mabou Tagne A et al, 'A Novel Standardized *Cannabis sativa* L. Extract and Its Constituent Cannabidiol Inhibit Human Polymorphonuclear Leukocyte Functions', *International Journal of Molecular Sciences,* 20, 8 (2019):1833

5 Appendino G et al, 'Antibacterial Cannabinoids from *Cannabis sativa*: A structure-activity study', *Journal of Natural Products*, 71, 8 (2008):1427–30

6 Pisanti S et al, 'CBD State of the Art and New Challenges for Therapeutic Applications', *Pharmacology and Therapeutics,* 175 (2017):133–150

7 Echo Pharma, 'Arvisol', echo-pharma.com, accessed 30 November 2019

8 Gibbs B et al, 'CBD in the UK: Executive summary', Centre for Medicinal Cannabis Report, 27 June 2019

4. How Hemp Is Grown for CBD

1 United Nations (1961), 'Single convention on narcotic drugs', unodc.org, accessed 30 November 2019

2 Gilbert A N, DiVerdi J A, 'Consumer Perceptions of

Strain Differences in Cannabis Aroma', *PLOS One*, 13, 2 (2018):e0192247

3 European Monitoring Centre for Drugs and Drug Addiction, 'Cannabis Legislation in Europe: An overview', Publications Office of the European Union, Luxembourg, corrected edition, June 2018

4 Sunstrand, 'Hemp: The Solution for Global Warming', sunstrands.com, 18 January 2019

5 Luo X et al, 'Complete Biosynthesis of Cannabinoids and Their Unnatural Analogues in Yeast', *Nature*, 567 (2019):123–126

5. How to Use CBD Safely

1 World Health Organization, 'Cannabidiol (CBD) Critical Review Report', Expert Committee on Drug Dependence, fortieth meeting, Geneva, 4–7 June 2018

2 Bonn-Miller M O et al, 'Labeling Accuracy of Cannabidiol Extracts Sold Online', *JAMA*, 318, 17 (2017):1708–1709

3 Gibbs B et al, 'CBD in the UK: Towards a responsible, innovative and high-quality cannabidiol industry', executive summary, Centre for Medicinal Cannabis, thecmcuk.org, 27 June 2019

4 Rianprakaisang T et al, 'Commercial Cannabidiol Oil Contaminated with the Synthetic Cannabinoid AB-FUBINACA Given to a Pediatric Patient', *Clinical Toxicology*, 24 May (2019):1

5 Xu J, 'You Can Now Buy CBD Oil Leggings, Here's What You Need to Know', bodyandsoul.com, 18 September 2019

6 Grant K S et al, 'Cannabis use during pregnancy: Pharmacokinetics and effects on child development', *Pharmacology and Therapeutics*, 182 (2018):133–151

7 World Anti-Doping Agency, 'Cannabinoid', wada-ama.org, accessed 30 November 2019

8 Corroon J, Phillips J A, 'A Cross-Sectional Study of Cannabidiol Users', *Cannabis and Cannabinoid Research*, 3, 1 (2018):152–161

9 Taylor L et al, 'A Phase I, Randomized, Double-blind, Placebo-controlled, Single Ascending Dose, Multiple Dose, and Food Effect Trial of the Safety, Tolerability and Pharmacokinetics of Highly Purified Cannabidiol in Healthy Subjects', *CNS Drugs,* 32, 11 (2018):1053–1067

10 'Army: 2 Deaths, 60 Hospitalizations Blamed on Vaping Oils', cbsnews.com, 1 February 2018
11 Poklis J L et al, 'The Unexpected Identification of the Cannabimimetic, 5F-ADB, and Dextromethorphan in Commercially Available Cannabidiol E-liquids', *Forensic Science International*, 294 (2019):e25–e27
12 Peace R M et al, 'Evaluation of Two Commercially Available Cannabidiol Formulations for Use in Electronic Cigarettes', *Frontiers in Pharmacology*, 7 (2016):279
13 Jensen R P et al, 'Hidden Formaldehyde in E-Cigarette Aerosols', *New England Journal of Medicine*, 372 (2015):392–394
14 Ogunwale M A et al, 'Aldehyde Detection in Electronic Cigarette Aerosols', *ACS Omega*, 2, 3 (2017):1207–1214

6. CBD For Pain and Other Physical Conditions

1 Fayaz A et al, 'Prevalence of Chronic Pain in the UK: A systematic review and meta-analysis of population studies', *BMJ Open*, 6, 6 (2016):e010364
2 British National Formulary, 'Non-steroidal Anti-Inflammatory Drugs. Therapeutic Effects', bnf.nice.org.uk, accessed 30 November 2019
3 Peter D Hart Research Associates, 'Americans Talk About Pain', researchamerica.org, August 2003
4 Russo E, 'Hemp for Headache: An in-depth historical and scientific review of cannabis in migraine treatment', *Journal of Cannabis Therapeutics*, 1, 2 (2001):21–91
5 Russo E, 'Clinical Endocannabinoid Deficiency Reconsidered: Current research supports the theory in migraine, fibromyalgia, irritable bowel, and other treatment-resistant syndromes', *Cannabis and Cannabinoid Research*, 1, 1 (2016):154–165
6 Troutt W D, DiDonato M D, 'Medical Cannabis in Arizona: Patient characteristics, perceptions, and impressions of medical cannabis legalization', *Journal of Psychoactive Drugs*, 47, 4 (2015):259–66
7 Whiting P F et al, 'Cannabinoids for Medical Use: A systematic review and meta-analysis', *JAMA*, 313, 24 (2015):2456–2473
8 Boehnke K F et al, 'High-Frequency Medical Cannabis Use Is Associated with Worse Pain among Individuals with Chronic Pain', *Journal of Pain*, (2019) pii: S1526–5900(19)30814–4

9   Wallace M et al, 'Dose-dependent Effects of Smoked Cannabis on Capsaicin-induced Pain and Hyperalgesia in Healthy Volunteers', *Anesthesiology*, 107, 5 (2007):785–96

10 Cunetti L et al, 'Chronic Pain Treatment with Cannabidiol in Kidney Transplant Patients in Uruguay', *Transplantation Proceedings*, 50, 2 (2018):461–464

11 Piermarini C, Viswanath O, 'CBD as the New Medicine in the Pain Provider's Armamentarium', *Pain and Therapy*, 8, 1 (2019):157–158

12 Bih C I et al, 'Molecular Targets of Cannabidiol in Neurological Disorders', *Neurotherapeutics*, 12, 4 (2015):699–730

13 Leimuranta P et al, 'Emerging Role of (Endo)Cannabinoids in Migraine', *Frontiers in Pharmacology*, 9 (2018): 420

14 Baron E P, 'Medicinal Properties of Cannabinoids, Terpenes, and Flavonoids in Cannabis, and Benefits in Migraine, Headache, And Pain: an update on current evidence and cannabis science', *Headache*, 58 (2018):1139–1186

15 Rhyne D N et al, 'Effects of Medical Marijuana on Migraine Headache Frequency in an Adult Population', *Pharmacotherapy*, 36 (2016):505–510

16 Nicolodi, et al, 'Cannabinoids Investigated for Treatment of Migraine' in 'Review of the 3rd European Academy of Neurology Congress 2017', *EMJ Neurology*, 5, 1 (2017):12–29

17 Russo E, 'Clinical Endocannabinoid Deficiency Reconsidered: Current Research Supports the Theory in Migraine, Fibromyalgia, Irritable Bowel, and Other Treatment-Resistant Syndromes', *Cannabis and Cannabinoid Research*, 1, 1 (2016):154–165

18 Camilleri M et al, 'Cannabinoid receptor 1 gene and irritable bowel syndrome: phenotype and quantitative traits', *American Journal of Physiology, Gastrointestinal And Liver Physiology*, 304 (2013):G553–G560

19 Di Carlo J, Izzo A A, 'Cannabinoids for Gastrointestinal Diseases: Potential therapeutic applications', *Expert Opinion on Investigational Drugs*, 12, 1 (2003):39–49; and Russo E B, 'Clinical Endocannabinoid Deficiency Reconsidered: Current research supports the theory in migraine, fibromyalgia, irritable bowel, and other treatment-resistant syndromes', *Cannabis and Cannabinoid Research*, 1, 1 (2016):154–165

20 Akbar A et al, 'Increased Capsaicin Receptor TRPV1-expressing Sensory Fibres in Irritable Bowel Syndrome

and their Correlation with Abdominal Pain', *Gut,* 57, 7 (2008):923–9

21 Esfandyari T et al, 'Effects of a Cannabinoid Receptor Agonist on Colonic Motor and Sensory Functions in Humans: A randomized, placebo-controlled study', *American Journal of Physiology, Gastrointestinal and Liver Physiology,* 293 (2007):G137–G145 5

22 Klooker T K et al, 'The Cannabinoid Receptor Agonist Delta-9-Tetrahydrocannabinol Does Not Affect Visceral Sensitivity to Rectal Distension in Healthy Volunteers and IBS Patients', *Neurogastroenterology and Motility,* 23 (2011):30–35, e2

23 Wong B S et al, 'Randomized Pharmacodynamic and Pharmacogenetic Trial of Dronabinol Effects on Colon Transit in Irritable Bowel Syndrome-Diarrhea', *Neurogastroenterology and Motility,* 24 (2012):358-e169

24 Harris R E, Clauw D J, 'Newer Treatments for Fibromyalgia Syndrome', *Therapeutics and Clinical Risk Management,* 4, 6 (2008):1331–42

25 Ross J, 'Pain 101: Looking to the Brain to Understand Fibromyalgia and Other Chronic Pain Conditions', relief.news, accessed 30 November 2019

26 Fitzcharles M A et al, 'Opioid Use in Fibromyalgia Is Associated with Negative Health Related Measures in a Prospective Cohort Study', *Pain Research and Treatment,* 2013, (2013):898493

27 Fiz J et al, 'Cannabis Use in Patients with Fibromyalgia: Effect on Symptoms Relief and Health-Related Quality of Life', *PLOS One,* 6, 4 (2011):e18440

28 Van de Donk T et al, 'An Experimental Randomized Study on the Analgesic Effects of Pharmaceutical-Grade Cannabis in Chronic Pain Patients with Fibromyalgia', *Pain,* 160, 4 (2019):860–869

29 National Institute for Health and Care Excellence, 'Scenario: Diverticular disease,' cks.nice.org.uk, March 2019

30 Guagnini F et al, 'Neural Contractions in Colonic Strips from Patients with Diverticular Disease: Role of endocannabinoids and substance P', *Gut,* 55, 7 (2006):946–53

31 Lahner E et al, 'High-fibre Diet and Lactobacillus Paracasei B21060 in Symptomatic Uncomplicated Diverticular Disease', *World Journal of Gastroenterology,* 18, 41 (2012):5918–24

32 Pariente B, Laharie D, 'Review Article: Why, when and how to de-escalate therapy in inflammatory bowel diseases', *Alimentary Pharmacology and Therapeutics*, 40 (2014):338–353

33 Alhamoruni A et al, 'Cannabinoids Mediate Opposing Effects on Inflammation-Induced Intestinal Permeability', *British Journal of Pharmacology*, 165, 8 (2012):2598–2610

34 Lal S et al, 'Cannabis Use amongst Patients with Inflammatory Bowel Disease', *European Journal of Gastroenterology and Hepatology*, 23, 10 (2011):891–6

35 Naftali T et al, 'Treatment of Crohn's Disease with Cannabis: An observational study', *Israel Medical Association Journal*, 13, 8 (2011):455–8

36 Irving P et al, 'A Randomized, Double-blind, Placebo-controlled, Parallel-group, Pilot Study of Cannabidiol-rich Botanical Extract in the Symptomatic Treatment of Ulcerative Colitis', *Inflammatory Bowel Diseases*, 24, 4 (2018):714–724

37 Naftali T et al, 'Low-dose Cannabidiol Is Safe but Not Effective in the Treatment for Crohn's Disease, a Randomized Controlled Trial', *Digestive Diseases and Sciences*, 62, 6 (2017):1615–1620

38 Armour M et al, 'Self-management Strategies amongst Australian Women with Endometriosis: A national online survey', *BMC Complementary and Alternative Medicine*, 19, 1 (2019):17

39 Sophocleous A et al, 'The Type 2 Cannabinoid Receptor Regulates Susceptibility to Osteoarthritis in Mice', *Osteoarthritis and Cartilage*, 23, 9 (2015):1586–94

40 Kuptniratsaikul V et al, 'Efficacy and Safety of Curcuma Domestica Extracts Compared with Ibuprofen in Patients with Knee Osteoarthritis: A multicenter study', *Clinical Interventions in Aging*, 9 (2014):451–8

41 Borsook D et al, 'Surgically-induced Neuropathic Pain (SNPP): Understanding the perioperative process', *Annals of Surgery*, 257, 3 (2013):403–412

42 Zhang J et al, 'Induction of CB2 Receptor Expression in the Rat Spinal Cord of Neuropathic But Not Inflammatory Chronic Pain Models', *European Journal of Neuroscience*, 17, 12 (2003):2750–4

43 Breivik H et al, 'Survey of Chronic Pain in Europe: Prevalence, impact on daily life, and treatment', *European Journal of Pain*, 10, 4 (2006):287–333

44 Rabgay K et al, 'The Effects of Cannabis, Cannabinoids,

and Their Administration Routes on Pain Control Efficacy and Safety: A systematic review and network meta-analysis', *Journal of the American Pharmacists Association*, (2019) pii: S1544–3191(19)30353-X

45 Casarette D J et al, 'Benefit of Tetrahydrocannabinol versus Cannabidiol for Common Palliative Care Symptoms', *Journal of Palliative Medicine*, 22, 10 (2019):1180–1184

46 Schleider L B L et al, 'Prospective Analysis of Safety and Efficacy of Medical Cannabis in Large Unselected Population of Patients with Cancer', *European Journal of Internal Medicine*, 49 (2018):37–43

47 Johnson J R et al, 'Multicenter, Double-blind, Randomized, Placebo-Controlled, Parallel-Group Study of the Efficacy, Safety, and Tolerability of THC:CBD Extract and THC Extract in Patients with Intractable Cancer-related Pain', *Journal of Pain and Symptom Management*, 39, 2 (2010):167–79

48 Johnson J R et al, 'An open-label extension study to investigate the long-term safety and tolerability of THC/ CB oromucosal spray and oromucosal THC spray in patients with terminal cancer-related pain refractory to strong opioid analgesics', *Journal of Pain and Symptom Management*, 46 (2013):207–218

49 Durst R et al, 'Cannabidiol, a Nonpsychoactive Cannabis Constituent, Protects against Myocardial Ischemic Reperfusion Injury', *American Journal of Physiology. Heart and Circulatory Physiology*, 293, 6 (2007):H3602–H3607

50 Pisanti S et al, 'CBD State of the Art and New Challenges for Therapeutic Applications', *Pharmacology and Therapeutics*, 175 (2017):133–150

51 Jadoon K A et al, 'A Single Dose of Cannabidiol Reduces Blood Pressure in Healthy Volunteers in a Randomized Crossover Study', *JCI Insight*, 2, 12 (2017) pii: 93760

52 Lee M J et al, 'The Effects of Hempseed Meal Intake and Linoleic Acid on Drosophila Models of Neurodegenerative Diseases and Hypercholesterolemia', *Molecules and Cells*, 31, 4 (2011):337–342

53 Bermúdez-Silva F J, 'Presence of Functional Cannabinoid Receptors in Human Endocrine Pancreas', *Diabetologia*, 51, 3 (2008):476–87

54 Weiss L et al, 'Cannabidiol Lowers Incidence of Diabetes in Non-obese Diabetic Mice', *Autoimmunity*, 39, 2 (2006):143–51

55 Smeriglio A et al, 'Inhibition of Aldose Reductase Activity

by *Cannabis sativa* Chemotypes Extracts with High Content of Cannabidiol or Cannabigerol', *Fitoterapia*, 127 (2018):101–108

56 Tiyerili V et al, 'CB1 Receptor Inhibition Leads to Decreased Vascular AT1 Receptor Expression, Inhibition of Oxidative Stress and Improved Endothelial Function', *Basic Research in Cardiology*, 105, 4 (2010):465–77

57 Hao E et al, 'Cannabidiol Protects against Doxorubicin-Induced Cardiomyopathy by Modulating Mitochondrial Function and Biogenesis', *Molecular Medicine*, 21 (2015):38–45

58 Rajesh M et al, 'Cannabidiol Attenuates Cardiac Dysfunction, Oxidative Stress, Fibrosis, Inflammatory and Cell Death Signaling Pathways in Diabetic Cardiomyopathy', *Journal of the American College of Cardiology*, 56, 25 (2010):2115–2125

59 El-Remessy A B et al, 'Cannabinoid 1 Receptor Activation Contributes to Vascular Inflammation and Cell Death in a Mouse Model of Diabetic Retinopathy and a Human Retinal Cell Line', *Diabetologia*, 54, 6 (2011):1567–78

60 Toth C C et al, 'Cannabinoid-mediated Modulation of Neuropathic Pain and Microglial Accumulation in a Model of Murine Type I Diabetic Peripheral Neuropathic Pain', *Molecular Pain*, 6 (2010):16

61 Lidell M E et al, 'Evidence for Two Types of Brown Adipose Tissue in Humans', *Nature Medicine*, 19 (2013):631–634

62 Kaisanlahti A, Glumoff T J, 'Browning of White Fat: Agents and implications for beige adipose tissue to type 2 diabetes', *Journal of Physiology and Biochemistry*, 75 (2019):1

63 Parray H A, Yun J W, 'Cannabidiol Promotes Browning in 3T3-L1 Adipocytes', *Molecular and Cellular Biochemistry*, 416 (2016):131

64 Le Foll B et al, 'The Future of endocannabinoid-oriented Clinical Research after CB1 Antagonists', *Psychopharmacology*, 205, 1 (2009):171–174

65 Juel-Jensen B E, 'Cannabis and Recurrent Herpes Simplex', *British Medical Journal*, 4, 5835 (1972):296

66 Morahan P S et al, 'Effects of Cannabinoids on Host Resistance to Listeria Monocytogenes and Herpes Simplex Virus', *Infection and Immunity*, 23, 3 (1979):670–4

67 Maor Y et al, 'Cannabidiol Inhibits Growth and Induces Programmed Cell Death in Kaposi Sarcoma-associated Herpesvirus-infected Endothelium', *Genes and Cancer*, 3, 7–8 (2012):512–20

68 Robinson E S et al, 'Knowledge, Attitudes, and Perceptions of Cannabinoids in the Dermatology Community', *Journal of Drugs in Dermatology,* 17, (2018):1273–1278

69 Wilkinson J D, Williamson E M, 'Cannabinoids Inhibit Human Keratinocyte Proliferation through a Non-CB1/CB2 Mechanism and Have a Potential Therapeutic Value in the Treatment of Psoriasis', *Journal of Dermatological Science*, 45, 2 (2007):87–92

70 Palmieri B et al, 'A Therapeutic Effect of CBD-enriched Ointment in Inflammatory Skin Diseases and Cutaneous Scars', *La Clinica Terapeutica*, 170, 2 (2019):e93–e99

71 Maida V, Corban J, 'Topical Medical Cannabis: A new treatment for wound pain – three cases of pyoderma gangrenosum', *Journal of Pain and Symptom Management*, 54, 5 (2017):732–736

72 Hammell D C et al, 'Transdermal Cannabidiol Reduces Inflammation and Pain-related Behaviours in a Rat Model of Arthritis', *European Journal of Pain,* 20, 6 (2016): 936–948

7. CBD For Emotional Wellbeing

1 Morena M et al, 'Neurobiological Interactions Between Stress and the Endocannabinoid System'. *Neuropsychopharmacology,* 41, 1 (2016):80–102

2 Hill M N, Patel S, 'Translational Evidence for the Involvement of the Endocannabinoid System in Stress-related Psychiatric Illnesses', *Biology of Mood and Anxiety Disorders*, 3, 1 (2013):19

3 Chouker A et al, 'Motion Sickness, Stress and the Endocannabinoid System', *PLOS One,* 5, 5 (2010):e10752

4 Elms L et al, 'Cannabidiol in the Treatment of Post-Traumatic Stress Disorder: A case series', *Journal of Alternative and Complementary Medicine*, 25, 4 (2019):392–397

5 Das R K et al, 'Cannabidiol Enhances Consolidation of Explicit Fear Extinction in Humans', *Psychopharmacology*, 226, 4 (2013):781–92

6 Soares V P, Campos A C, 'Evidences for the Anti-panic Actions of Cannabidiol', *Current Neuropharmacology*, 15, 2 (2017):291–299

7 Christensen R et al, 'Efficacy and Safety of the Weight-loss Drug Rimonabant: A meta-analysis of randomised trials', *Lancet,* 370, 9600 (2007):1706–13

8 Zuardi A W et al, 'Action of Cannabidiol on the Anxiety and Other Effects Produced by Delta 9-THC in Normal Subjects', *Psychopharmacology*, 76 (1982):245–50

9 Zuardi A W et al, 'Effects of Ipsapirone and Cannabidiol on Human Experimental Anxiety', *Journal of Psychopharmacology*, 7 (1993):82–8

10 Bergamaschi M M et al, 'Cannabidiol Reduces the Anxiety Induced by Simulated Public Speaking in Treatment-naïve Social Phobia Patients', *Neuropsychopharmacology*, 36, 6 (2011):1219–26

11 Crippa J A et al, 'Effects of Cannabidiol (CBD) on Regional Cerebral Blood Flow', *Neuropsychopharmacology*, 29, 2 (2004):417–26

12 Fusar-Poli P, 'Distinct Effects of D9-tetrahydrocannabinol and Cannabidiol on Neural Activation During Emotional Processing', *Archives of General Psychiatry*, 66, 1 (2009): 95–105

13 Shannon S et al, 'Cannabidiol in Anxiety and Sleep: A large case series', *Permanente Journal*, 23 (2019):18–041

14 Schier A R et al, 'Cannabidiol, a *Cannabis sativa* Constituent, As an Anxiolytic Drug', *Brazilian Journal of Psychiatry*, 34, Suppl 1 (2012):S104–10

15 Sales A J et al, 'Cannabidiol Induces Rapid and Sustained Antidepressant-like Effects Through Increased BDNF Signaling and Synaptogenesis in the Prefrontal Cortex', *Molecular Neurobiology*, 56, 2 (2019):1070–1081

16 Vaughn L K et al, 'Endocannabinoid Signalling: Has it got rhythm?', *British Journal of Pharmacology*, 160, 3 (2010):530–43

17 Babson K A et al, 'Cannabis, Cannabinoids, and Sleep: a Review of the Literature', *Current Psychiatry Reports*, 19, 4 (2017):23

18 Ibid.

19 Carlini E A, Cunha J M, 'Hypnotic and Antiepileptic Effects of Cannabidiol', *Journal of Clinical Pharmacology*, 21, S1 (1981):417S–427S

20 Shannon S et al, 'Cannabidiol in Anxiety and Sleep: A large case series', *Permanente Journal*, 23 (2019):18–041

21 Daniells S, 'Seminal Findings: First report of safety and efficacy of hemp-derived, CBD-rich extract in healthy humans', nutraingredients-USA.com, 21 June 2019

22 Morgan C et al, 'Cannabidiol Attenuates the Appetitive Effects of δ9-tetrahydrocannabinol in Humans Smoking

References

Their Chosen Cannabis', *Neuropsychopharmacology*, 35, 9 (2010):1879–85

23   Morgan C J et al, 'Cannabidiol Reduces Cigarette Consumption in Tobacco Smokers: Preliminary findings', *Addictive Behaviors*, 38, 9 (2013):2433–6

8. Hemp Seed Oil

1   Bosy T Z, Cole K A, 'Consumption and Quantitation Of Delta9-tetrahydrocannabinol in Commercially Available Hemp Seed Oil Products', *Journal of Analytical Toxicology*, 24, 7 (2000):562–6

2   Petrovic M et al, 'Relationship Between Cannabinoids Content and Composition of Fatty Acids in Hempseed Oils', *Food Chemistry*, 170 (2015):218–25

3   Callaway J et al, 'Efficacy of Dietary Hempseed Oil in Patients with Atopic Dermatitis', *Journal of Dermatological Treatment*, 16, 2 (2005):87–94

4   Rezapour-Firouzi S et al, 'Erythrocyte Membrane Fatty Acids in Multiple Sclerosis Patients and Hot-nature Dietary Intervention with Co-Supplemented Hemp-Seed and Evening-Primrose Oils', *African Journal of Traditional Complementary and Alternative Medicines*, 10, 6 (2013):519–527

9. PEA – The New CBD Alternative

1   Jonsson K O et al, 'Effects of Homologues and Analogues of Palmitoylethanolamide upon the Inactivation of the Endocannabinoid Anandamide', *British Journal of Pharmacology*, 133, 8 (2001):1263–75

2   Artukoglu B B et al, 'Efficacy of Palmitoylethanolamide for Pain: A meta-analysis', *Pain Physician*, 20, 5 (2017):353–362

3   Paladini A et al, 'Palmitoylethanolamide, a Special Food for Medical Purposes, in the Treatment of Chronic Pain: A pooled data meta-analysis', *Pain Physician*, 19, 2 (2016):11–24

4   Steels E et al, 'A Double-blind Randomized Placebo Controlled Study Assessing Safety, Tolerability and Efficacy of Palmitoylethanolamide for Symptoms of Knee Osteoarthritis', *Inflammopharmacology*, 27, 3 (2019):475–485

5   Evangelista M et al, 'Ultra-micronized Palmitoylethanolamide Effects on Sleep-wake Rhythm

and Neuropathic Pain Phenotypes in Patients with Carpal Tunnel Syndrome: An open-label, randomized controlled study', *CNS And Neurological Disorders Drug Targets*, 17, 4 (2018):291–298

6 Hauer D et al, 'Plasma Concentrations of Endocannabinoids and Related Primary Fatty Acid Amides in Patients with Post-traumatic Stress Disorder', *PLOS One*, 8, 5 (2013):e62741

7 Yuan C et al, 'N-palmitoylethanolamine and N-acetylethanolamine Are Effective in Asteatotic Eczema: Results of a randomized, double-blind, controlled study in 60 patients', *Clinical Interventions in Aging*, 9 (2014):1163–9

8 Petrosini S, Di Marzo V, 'The Pharmacology of Palmitoylethanolamide and First Data on the Therapeutic Efficacy of Some of its New Formulations', *British Journal of Pharmacology*, 174, 11 (2017):1349–1365

Index

(Page numbers in *italic* refer to diagrams)

Index

Index

Index

Index

Index

premenstrual hormone tension (PMT), 144
prescription opioids, 9
prescriptions, 33
private clinics, 31, 33-4
probiotics, 150, 160, 166-7
Prohibition, 27, 51
prohibition, 5, 27, 51
Project 2021, 34
propylene glycol, 95, 117
prostaglandins, 65, 139, 249
prostate pain, 111
pruritus, 202
psoriasis, 64, 71, 169, 202-5, 214, 249,
psoriatic arthritis, 69, 169
psychoactive, 1–4, 6, 17, 22–5, 28, 46, 49, 54, 62, 66, 67, 72, 77, 81, 97, 102, 118, 175, 262
psychoactive effects, described, 24
psychoactive 'high,' 2
psychosis, 39, 46, 62, 71, 210
PTSD, 34, *71*, 210, 213, 220–1, 256
purification, 94–5

qunabu, 3

Radcliffe Infirmary, Oxford, 199
radioactive waste, 54, 86
Raleigh, Sir Walter, 27
rapid eye movement, *see* REM
rapid pulse, 156
reasons for use, 8–9
rebound headache, 129
receptors, 56–9 (*see also by name*)
recreational marijuana, 36–7, 40, 137
    defined, 19, 265
rectal suppositories, 111
refractory pain, 133

Register of Nutrition and Health Claims (EU), 105, 121
regulations, *see* Good Manufacturing Practice
relaxation, 4
REM (rapid eye movement), 155, 238–42, 255
research, 50–1
restlessness, 210, 241
rheumatoid arthritis, 64, 68, 69, 71, 124, 133, 169, 172, 249, 251, 254
Rhodiola rosea, 121
rice, 12
Rimonabant, 50, 196-7, 228
rosin, 33
'rubbing it better,' 201
rubs, *see* topicals

safety, 9–11, 96–119
St John's wort, 121
salt intake, 182
Samaritans, 48, 234, 268
Scandinavia, 82
scavenger cells, 57, 202
scent, 77–9
Schedule 1 drugs, 6, 30, 36, 90, 146Schedule 2 drugs, 30
schizophrenia, 71
scleroderma, 50, 68
second brain, 151–2
Second World War, 4, 90
seizures, 25, 27, 46, 47, 60, 71, 117
selective serotonin reuptake inhibitors (SSRIs), *see* SSRIs
self-offsetting, 85
Selye, Dr Hans, 210
serotonin, 65, 131, 138, 139, 144, 151, 196, 216, 221, 231, 232, 235, 236
sexual activity, 144, 167, 214, 249
Shen Nung, 25